HARDCORE HEALTH: LIVE YOUNG!

ROBERT YONOVER PhD
ADAM CROWE PDC
JENNIFER ARMSTRONG MS, MD.

Recipes by Katie Amato, MA Public Health
Illustrations by Janet King

© Copyright 2019 Beacon Publishing Group
All rights reserved.

No portion of this book may be reproduced in whole or in part, by any means whatsoever, except for passages excerpted for the purposes of review, without the prior written permission of the publisher. For information, or to order additional copies, please contact:

Beacon Publishing Group
P.O. Box 41573 Charleston, S.C. 29423
800.817.8480| beaconpublishinggroup.com

Publisher's catalog available by request.

ISBN-13: 978-1-949472-61-5

ISBN-10: 1-949472-61-2

Published in 2019. New York, NY 10001.

First Edition. Printed in the USA.

Foreword—Dr. Joseph Pizzorno ND..............**i**
PART 1—LIVE YOUNG, AN INVENTOR'S BLUEPRINT
Introduction—Robert Yonover PhD...................1
Chapter 1—Physical Diet...........................**5**
    Diet for a Healthy You.........................5
    Dr. Rob's Push-button Diet..................10
    Water...17
    Poop Watch......................................18
    Exercise..**21**
    High and Low Impact Sports................22
    To Train or Not to Train.....................24
    Walking...26
    Biking...28
    Paddle/Dive Swim.............................29
    One-Breath Free Dives......................32
    Rough Water Swim...........................34
    Paddle/Belly Ride.............................36
    Maintenance....................................38
    Staying Fit in the City.......................39
    Your Skin And Non-Surgical Solutions To Make You Look Youthful—Jennifer Armstrong MS, MD, Advanced Skincare Surgery and Medcenter, Newport Beach CA...43
    Protect Your Skin.............................43
    Get That Glow.................................44
    Reduce Skin Damage........................45
    Prevent Aging..................................45
    Non-surgical Solutions.......................45

Restoring Volume to Your Face............46
Soften Wrinkles and Crow's feet under
Eyes...46
Soften Lines around Lips.....................47
Stimulate Collagen............................47
Botox Neck Lift...............................48
Solutions for Sun Damage on Chest........49
Solutions for Acne and Oily Skin..........49
Solutions for Large Pores, Skin tone, and
texture...50
Hair...50
Washing...50
New Ways to Fight Baldness.................51
Teeth..54
Supplements....................................55
Mild Semi-Natural Stimulants............59
Sex..61
Love and Health..............................61
Keep Things Flowing........................62
Kegel Exercises for Men and Women......62
Nitric Oxide and Sex........................66
Viagra and Other Medications..............69
Sexy Foods....................................69
Physical Labor................................76
Rehab..77
Sleep As Fuel.................................78
Sleep Sabotages..............................81
Perpetual Working.........................84
Chapter 2—Fight Disease With Diet And Lifestyle...87

Fight Cancer With Diet And Lifestyle...87
    Fight Prostate Cancer.........................90
    Fight Colon Cancer............................94
    Fight Lung Cancer.............................96
    Fight Breast Cancer...........................99
    Fight Skin Cancer............................103
    Dangerous Moles.............................108
Fight Diabetes With Diet And Lifestyle……………………………...109
    Eliminate Toxins..............................109
    Maintain a Healthy Weight.................110
Fight Heart Disease With Diet And Lifestyle……………………………...114
    Symptoms of a Heart Attack...............117
    Warning Signs of a Stroke..................118
    Key Nutrient Deficiencies..................120
    Foods to Avoid...............................121
Chapter 3—Mental................................126
    Goals and a Sense of Purpose.............126
    Brain Health...................................129
    What Helps Your Brain?....................130
    What Hurts Your Brain?....................131
    Keep Your Mind Fit.........................134
    Brain Food....................................135
    Positive Pessimism—A Form of Optimism.....................................136
    Balance..137
    Take a Break.................................139
    Reward Yourself.............................141
Chapter 4—Social..................................144

    Family………………………………..144
    Kids…………………………………..145
    Friends and Clubs……………………147
    Human Interaction and the
    Smartphone…………………………..153
    Solitude……………………………….154

Chapter 5—Spiritual………………………….156
    Nature………………………………....156
    Music………………………………….157
    Religion……………………………….158
    Service and Giving Back……………..159

PART 2—LIVING CLOSE TO NATURE
    Introduction—Adam Crowe PDC………160

Chapter 6—You Are What You Breathe, Drink And Eat…………………………………………...164
    Primary Elements……………………..164
    Air……………………………………..166
    Water………………………………….168
    Fire (Sunlight)………………………...172
    Earth…………………………………..174
    Your Digestive System and Staying
    Young………………………………...181

Chapter 7—How To Grow Your Own………..186
    Reasons to Grow Your Own…………..186
    Sprouting……………………………...187
    How to Sprout Seeds…………………..188
    Balcony and Patio Herb Garden………..190
    Backyard Gardens……………………..193
    Garden Beds…………………………..193

Good Soil………………………………….194
Trellising………………………………….. 196
What to Grow and When to Grow It……197
Spring—Cool Season Crops……………199
Summer—Warm Season Crops………...199

PART 3—WHOLESOME, DELICIOUS RECIPES FROM KATIE'S TROPICAL KITCHEN

Introduction—Katie Amato M.A. Public Health……………………………………...200
Beverages: Drink Your Vitamins……….201
Smoothies……………………………….201
Juices……………………………………..203
Salad and Side dishes…………………...207
Light Meals……………………………..214
Main Meals……………………………..226
Healthy Desserts………………………...240

"It's been an honor and a pleasure to surf the big waves of the North Shore with Dr. Yonover. Knowing your own physical fitness and confidence is one of your most important survival tools out there. This book is a must have for those that want to stay fit and confident in their bodies to keep in the game!"
-Clay Everline, M.D. Author of Surf Survival (now in its second edition)

"Life is so short; why not start feeling better today? This is a wonderful all-inclusive book on health. It's easy to read, fun, funny and extremely educational. I highly recommend it to anyone ready to kick-start a healthy life right now. I completely agree with Dr. Rob that our bodies are meant to be flexible and strong well into our senior years, and that proper diet and exercise are the key ingredients. In a light-hearted way, Dr. Rob prescribes easy and fun lifestyle changes. This is a must-read for all who are serious about truly enjoying life."
- Renee Linnell, surfer, snowboarder, ex-professional dancer, and author of The Burn Zone: a Memoir

"At 48 years old and 240 pounds I decided to change my life by following Dr. Yonover's program. In only 1 year, I lost 55 pounds and I've never felt better or stronger. Dr. Yonover's methods work!"
-Darren C. Blum, Retired Attorney.

FOREWORD—Dr. Joseph E. Pizzorno, ND

We seem to be bifurcating as a society into those who learn about how to be healthy and take care of themselves and those who choose instead to simply live the commercialized low-nutrient, high-toxin, sedentary lifestyle. Since you are reading this book, I suspect you are one of the former. I very much enjoy reading and learning from others, such as Robert Yonover Ph.D. and Adam Crowe, who have dedicated their lives to solving the challenge of how to live a full and healthy life with little or no disease.

I have been involved in medicine now for almost half a century: as a researcher in conventional medicine, naturopathic medical student, naturopathic physician, teacher, prolific author, founding president of Bastyr University and advocate for natural medicine at the local, state, national and international levels.

When I chose to make the risky life choice to leave conventional medicine to become a naturopathic doctor, I had to take a lot on faith. It seemed logical to me that health depended upon eating real food, avoiding toxins, being physically active and having loving relationships. However, not only was there little research support, the conventional world vigorously discounted these ideas and discredited anyone who would presume to suggest that diet and lifestyle were important to health. (Please don't believe the conventional medicine apologists who now assert MDs always thought these were important. During most of the 20th century they aggressively did everything they could to outlaw natural medicine. Many of my teachers were jailed for telling their patients to eat healthfully rather than take drugs. MDs appeared in cigarette ads asserting that smoking was not bad for people. In the 1970s, I had several very contentious debates with an MD researcher who argued vociferously that "Food does not affect you. The average diet is totally healthy." I could go on…)

Over these 5 decades, I have taught thousands of students and doctors, authored or co-authored 12 books and textbooks (newest is *The Toxin Solution),* written over 100 articles in scientific journals and cared for tens of thousands of patients either directly or indirectly through sophisticated corporate wellness programs I designed and helped implement. During this time— despite huge investment in conventional medicine research and healthcare— we have seen a relentless increase in virtually all chronic diseases in all age groups. Clearly, something is wrong.

Research now conclusively documents that what you eat, how you live, and the toxins you let into your body have a huge effect on your susceptibility to disease. In fact, only 20% of disease is due to genetics, the rest is up to you. Not only have the guidelines to healthy living presented in this book been shown effective, but having practiced this myself virtually my whole life, I have had direct personal experience watching what happened to my friends and family according to the choices they made.

I am an avid basketball player (sorry Rob!) and have been playing with the same group of guys for almost 30 years. Or perhaps I should say I have been playing at the same gym these 3 decades because almost everyone in my age decade and the decade younger is now no longer playing. They lived the standard unhealthy American diet and lifestyle, took nonsteroidal anti-inflammatory drugs for the soreness after playing 1-2 hours of full court ball (yes Rob, basketball is a traumatic game) and often went out for a beer or three after the game. By age 50-55, virtually every one drops out as their bodies have simply broken down. Now I play with new guys who are half my age, and really enjoy when each eventually pulls me aside to ask, "How old are you?!"

My wife Lara and I have also watched what happened to our friends and family. We are now well past the so-called retirement age and still going strong with little disease. But so many of our friends and family are now either dead, suffering from multiple chronic diseases, or done with life. I took a photo at Lara's alumnae reunion a year ago, where classmates (who were still alive and able) gathered to meet up 45 years after graduation. Looking at the picture, you'd think my wife was the daughter of one of her past classmates.

Why the difference? We live a life very similar to the guidance you will read here.

Your choice: do you want a shorter life burdened with disease and fatigue? Or do you want a life of vitality and adventure? The choice is yours.

Joseph Pizzorno ND

Dr. Joseph Pizzorno, one of the world's leading authorities on science-based natural medicine, was appointed by President Clinton in December 2000 to the White House Commission on Complementary and Alternative Medicine Policy and by the President Bush's administration to the Medicare Coverage Advisory Committee in November 2002. Dr. Pizzorno is founding president of Bastyr University, Editor-in-Chief of Integrative Medicine: A Clinician's Journal, a member of the scientific review board of the Gateway for Cancer Research and Vice-chair of the Board of Directors of the Institute for Functional Medicine. Recipient of numerous awards and honors for his academic, professional and public affairs leadership, Dr. Pizzorno is the co-author of the internationally acclaimed Textbook of Natural Medicine, the best-selling Encyclopedia of Natural Medicine (2,000,000 copies in six languages), The Toxin Solution and 10 other books.

Hardcore Health: Live Young!

PART 1—LIVE YOUNG, AN INVENTOR'S BLUEPRINT

INTRODUCTION

As a lifelong inventor and scientist, I believe the number one eternal challenge is how to beat old age. *Hardcore Health: Live Young!* represents an inventor's perspective on how to attack and solve the problem of aging by staying healthy and living young.

Modern medicine has found ways to prolong life. Scientists say some babies born today will live to 104. According to the latest Census Bureau statistics, there are 53,364 centenarians in the U.S. today and experts estimate that number will rise to 600,000 by 2050. But what about the quality of life? We don't just want to live. We want to live young. We want to enjoy life, be active, look good, travel, make love and socialize. Bathing in the blood of virgins didn't work when Katherine the Great tried it. What will?

I come from a long line of still healthy survivors. My grandmother came to the U.S. by boat from Europe after her seven brothers left her there fearing she could not make the journey (and she was a bit of a pain in the ass). She told them to screw off and came anyway on her own, arriving in the U.S. in the early 1900's. She became one of the first female medical doctors and lived to 90+ years old. She was role model number one as she told us young ones to eat our "vege-tables."

Role model number two is my father, her son, who survived The Great Depression, got a Purple Heart in the Battle of the Bulge at the age of 18, and continues to be an inspiration as a physical specimen at the age of 93 and still going strong. To this day, he continues to eat a work lunch of fresh cut vegetables and fruit self-packed in a kid's school plastic lunch box.

Role model number three is Louie Zamperini, an Olympic athlete, who survived 47 days lost at sea in a raft, followed by two years of torture in a POW camp in World War II (see book and movie *Unbroken*).

Louie told me that one of his anti-aging secrets is also based on a fruit, however it comes from people stepping on them to make grapes into wine——his grandmother told him to drink a glass of red wine every day and it worked. Not only did it help his tortured internal organs recover after his POW stint, it enabled him to still keep active at the age of 97!

The "will to survive" also speaks to the mental capacity people have to survive horrible situations. Louie told me that there was no way those torturous POW prison guards were going to break him—especially after he'd survived an airplane ditching in the ocean and 47 days in a raft!

Hardcore Health: Live Young!

Another hero of mine is General William Spruance, an aviator horribly injured in a plane crash, who was able to survive and share his experience and philosophies well into his 90's, including the process of having his arm sewn into an opening in his stomach for months to aid in the healing of his burns! When I met the General it was hard to look at his disfigured body and burned skin; however, as he shared his story, the scars became lifetime achievement awards (tattoos) in my mind. While talking to both these men, I realized that however hard you may think a situation is, it is probably nowhere near as drastic as what they went through and survived!

As a scientist and inventor, I have always been obsessed with problem solving, especially if it relates to problems that I personally want to tackle. One of the problems I really wanted to solve was being lost at sea or in the wild. That's why I invented the See/Rescue Streamer, emergency survival equipment. It is also why I invented the Inflatable Paddleboard, a paddleboard I can check as baggage on a plane or pack in a suitcase. See my book Hardcore Inventing for further details.

Another problem I really would like to solve, and I'm sure you would too, is aging. The problem, for me, is twofold:

1. I really don't like doctors and/or being sick.

2. I am extremely competitive and don't want to miss out on any fun activities in life, especially a good swell on the North Shore. (Note that I am a black-tar surfing addict.)

Having witnessed my four role models, my grandmother, dad, Louie, and the General in action, I combined their input with the explosion of information at our fingertips on the internet and news media and devised a multitude of techniques and skills to optimize my personal aging. *Hardcore Health: Live Young*! shares those techniques for you to incorporate into your life so you can optimize your existence and chase down your own personal dreams and aspirations.

Enjoy! Stay Hardcore! Live Young!!!!
Robert Yonover PhD

CHAPTER 1—PHYSICAL

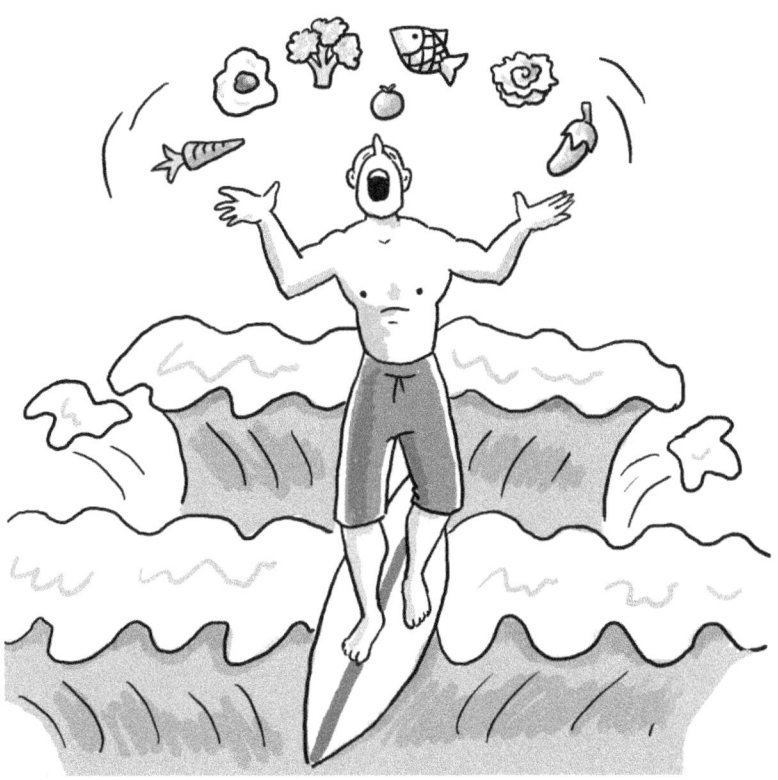

DIET FOR A HEALTHY YOU

As an inventor of survival gear, I try to solve the problem at hand with the least amount of materials in the least amount of time— like your life depends on it and you have a clock counting down before you're going to die, as in real life

MacGyver situations. Nature is the other driving force of my inventions. I look to nature for inspiration and insight, as all living creatures continue to evolve to survive.

Diet is no different. I consider myself an aquatic ape or water-ape and try to think in a primitive ape-like manner. As humans, I don't think we were meant to gorge on the food that many people eat now; food that results in horrific obesity and related illness, namely heart attacks, strokes and diabetes. Perhaps if we all ran around naked with full-length mirrors and weighing scales surrounding us, we would take better care of ourselves. And we might finally realize that it is critical to eat well if you want to live well.

When primitive humans ran around the earth, there were no fast food places serving junk food and soda. I am fortunate enough to have traveled to Africa and seen how wild animals live. Wild animals have an extremely low rate of success at killing prey. Because of this, they scrounge around on scraps until they make a kill every few days or weeks. This is my basic philosophy on eating meat. I don't have it in my fridge and only occasionally make a kill at a remote restaurant location.

A study supported by the NIH's National Health, Lung and Blood Institute (NHLBI), National Cancer Institute (NCI) and National Institute of Diabetes and Digestive and Kidney diseases (NIDDK) found that those who consumed the highest levels of both unprocessed and processed red meat have the highest risk of cancer mortality and cardiovascular mortality. See Archives of Internal Medicine on March 12, 2012. https://www.nih.gov/news-events/nih-research-matters/risk-red-meat. Also, diabetes prevalence increased as the frequency of meat consumption increased. (See the following website: https://www.ncbi.nlm.nih.gov/pmc/articles/PMC3942738.)

Substituting one serving per day of foods like fish, legumes, poultry, low-fat dairy, nuts and whole grains could lower this risk. Scientists calculated 9.3% of deaths in men and 7.6% of women could have been prevented if the participants had consumed fewer than half a serving per day (about 1.5 ounces) of red meat.

I am essentially a beanatarian with a superfood/fuel addiction (see my Push Button Super Fuel Diet below, a.k.a. beans, greens and proteins with a colon blow twist). Food is expensive and critical to your health, so why not buy, catch and consume the best food you can, the less processed the better. I believe you should be cutting up raw food like vegetables or breaking up plants like cabbage with your bare hands. Of course, there is a green aspect to this technique as I try to eat locally grown foods. My main staples consist of locally grown Japanese eggplant and cabbage.

A parallel principle is the "colon-blow" philosophy and for this I credit a Saturday Night Live skit of 20+ years ago on moving volume. Our bodies are our temples or in this case our factories, and we have to move a lot of product through to remain vibrant. Along those same lines, if you take in a high-fiber super fuel diet 80% of the time, the other 20% of the time you can eat anything, and this is where I get my meat intake. I call this the 80-20 rule and it seems to work. If you mix in a little junk food with your premium, massive-volume, super-fuel diet, your digestive system laughs at the imposters and moves them right along!

If you are not close to your food source in your cave, you can always venture out to stores if you have to. When buying food off the shelf, make sure you read the labels. There are two keys in my mind:

Fat Content: Make sure the calories from fat are 30% or less of the total calories. To make this determination, simply multiply the grams of fat x 9 and then divide it into the total calories. For example: Label reads: Total calories – 150, Fat – 5 grams. Multiply 5 grams x 9 = 45. 45/150 = ~30%. Memorize this simple formula and it will enable you to avoid purchasing highly fattening foods.

Net Carb Content: Make sure your net carb (carbohydrate) amount is as low as possible. I have a generic rule to start with: "avoid the color white," as I consider most processed food white or any food made by someone in a white coat. Eat the most primitive grains you can. I use a cut off of 3 grams of fiber or more. Note that brown rice is only 2 grams of fiber, so it no longer makes my cut. Same with breads— make sure you get bread that is at least 3 grams of fiber, preferably 5 grams or more. When reading labels, the other key is "Net Carbs" and that number should be as low as possible. Examples: White bread or crackers are 30+ Grams Carbs – 1 gram of Fiber = 29 Net Carbs. All Bran Cereal: 13 Grams Carbs – 11 Grams Fiber = 2 Net Carbs! By adding mega-fiber grains to the mix (All Bran and flax seed, see below), the effect is a very healthy Net Carb/High Fiber colon-blow concoction, with a hearty taste!

Note that regardless of how high in fiber the carb may be, you should still try to minimize your total carb input. For example, I recently cut my cereal portion to half a bowl and only one piece of bread per day with the immediate results noticeable in my overall health. I basically treat all carbs as a special treat and that includes the only no fiber carb that makes my cut— chocolate.

Below are meals from my Push Button Super Fuel Diet (not for the faint of heart), a.k.a. beans, greens, and proteins with a colon blow twist. This is the diet that makes me feel great. I'd eat it every day if my wife and kids would allow. The effectiveness of eating this way could be summed up in the phrase "the proof is in the pudding," however in this case you want to eat right so there is no pudding on your body when you look in the mirror, and that is the proof!

Dr. Rob's Push Button Super Fuel Breakfast
All-Bran Flakes, Buds
Flax Seed (3 teaspoonfuls) (Note: I now have to recommend this only for women as they have found that there are estrogen-like properties in Flax Seed and that is a non-starter for me as I want to remain as macho as possible.)
Almond Milk
Alternate occasionally with three egg and mushroom omelet

Dr. Rob's Push Button Super Fuel Lunch
Appetizer:
1 handful walnuts, almonds, cashews
1/2 teaspoon of cinnamon (washed down with water)
1/4 teaspoon of turmeric (washed down with water)
1 tablespoon chia seeds
1 tablespoon hemp seed hearts

Lunch Plate 1
Hulless Barley (Make in Rice Cooker, extra water just like cooking brown rice. Buy at Health Food Store).

Hardcore Health: Live Young!

Veggie Chili on top or Madras Indian Curry with Lentils and Red Beans is best for me, but anything with beans.

I have actually upped the ante and now make my own 7-Bean Indian Curry in the Crock Pot (see below) and just leave it in the fridge and scoop out servings from there.

Lunch Plate 2
Japanese Eggplant (Steamed)
Shredded cheese top off and cook together or let it melt as it cools off.

Lunch Plate 3
Cabbage (raw, break up and eat like lettuce)
Italian dressing or avocado oil/olive oil and balsamic vinegar with parmesan cheese

Dessert
1 small handful each of almonds, walnuts and cashews
4 small bites of dark chocolate morsels alternating with four spoonfuls of coconut oil. (My version of the healthy man's Mounds Bar®.)

Dr. Rob's Push Button Super Fuel Ginger Tea Time
Slice a half-fist size of fresh ginger root (buy in bulk at store). Boil sliced ginger with water. Let sit for 5 minutes and occasionally stab or squeeze

pieces of ginger. Pour the ginger/water through a strainer into an insulated mug. Add hot water for hot tea or cold water for iced tea.

Dr. Rob's Push Button Super Fuel Dinner (Eat as early as possible)
    Option 1. Veggie Burger or salmon burger (from Costco) with high fiber multi-grain bread (open-face, one piece only)
    Option 2. Hummus on top of Veggie-Burger, brown mustard on top of salmon burger
    Option 3. Egg and Spinach Greek omelet
    Option 4. Tuna (with mayo/relish) with high fiber (5 grams or more) multi-grain bread (open-face, one piece only)
    Plate covered with one of the following steamed veggies: Broccoli, spinach, asparagus, kale, collard greens, brussel sprouts or any mixture of the above. Add shredded cheese as it cools. Alternate 1 through 4 above for variation.

    Dessert
    1 handful pecans, macadamia nuts
    4 small bites of dark chocolate morsels.

RECIPES
Dr. Rob's Push Button Super Fuel Seven Bean Indian Curry
    Get a large crock pot.
    Add the following:

Hardcore Health: Live Young!

5.5 cups diced tomatoes
1 cup almond milk
1/4 stick butter
1/2 teaspoon salt
1/2 teaspoon pepper
1 teaspoon chili pepper flakes
3 teaspoons curry powder (get the good stuff from an Indian or health food store: either regular golden or "Madras" curry powder)
3 teaspoons garlic
Stir it all up
(Use dry beans from health food store bins or grocery store, wash/soak as desired)
1/2 cup garbanzo beans
1/2 cup brown lentils
1/2 cup red lentils
1/2 cup navy beans
1/2 cup red beans
1/2 cup lima beans
1/2 cup northern beans or any other white bean
Stir it all up
2 sliced up large onions
4 sliced up large carrots, the thicker the better
Add water to the top of the crock pot so it is almost spilling over. Stir it all up. Place newspaper under the crock-pot for spillage. Simmer on low for nine hours. Turn off and let sit for four hours. Stir occasionally. Place in fridge and scoop out and

reheat as needed. Place on top of hulless barley, sprinkle a little cheese and add some chili pepper flakes to your taste. GRIND!!!

Dr. Rob's Blackened Fish (or Chicken/Veggies)

My quick go-to preparation for fish revolves around a cast-iron skillet. I was on a flight years ago and a Cajun woman from New Orleans shared her blackening secrets. First and foremost, you have to "season" the pan by putting oil in it and baking it in the oven for several hours, a few times if you can.

Her other secret is that you never wash a cast-iron skillet, just wipe off the old oil with a paper towel and then re-oil it with fresh oil and store it wet with oil until your next use. A few years ago, I went to a party and brought my cast-iron skillet along with some fresh fish I caught to do it right for the revelers. A huge success, however I wasn't guarding my skillet and the host of the party washed my pan with soap and water— after over 10 years of cumulative seasoning/blackening on that pan (the more seasoning, the better the fish) — I am still mad to this day, more at myself for not keeping track of it than at him for washing it.

In regard to the oil, I recently switched from vegetable oil to avocado oil. Avocado oil is healthy and can still achieve the high temperatures, without burning, required for blackening.

Here is the basic step-by-step procedure:

Hardcore Health: Live Young!

1. Put cast-iron skillet with (avocado) oil on burner set to high. Heat for 10 minutes, continuing to oscillate the oil around the pan so it does not become dry and burn.
2. Sprinkle blackening spice (I prefer Chef Paul Prudhomme's "Blackened Redfish Magic" in red and white container) on fish fillets (or chicken or vegetables).
3. Place fillets with seasoned side down on the hot skillet.
4. Sprinkle up-side of fillets with additional spice.
5. Watch closely and flip the fillets within minutes (or seconds if you want just a quick flash-blackening with raw fish in the middle. This is ideal for fresh caught ahi (yellow fin tuna).
6. Mix shoyu (soy sauce) and wasabi (green spicy Japanese mustard) into a light paste.
7. Dip blackened fish in the shoyu and wasabi sauce and prepare for nirvana.
8. If using fresh-frozen fish, I usually make an open-face sandwich or a fish burrito.

Dr. Lava's Secret BBQ Marinade (a.k.a. "Rob's Fish").

Forty plus years ago, I created a BBQ marinade with a lucky combination of a several ingredients. It makes fish taste like steak and everyone who has tried it still raves about it. It also turns kids that hate fish into fish lovers (I lie to them at first and tell them it is chicken or steak). I've kept the recipe secret for years, but I think I am ready to share it. Check in at www.HardcoreInventing.com for details.

For more recipes, go to PART 3 for Wholesome and Delicious Recipes from Katie's Tropical Kitchen.

Legumes

Look into legumes as a healthy addition to your diet. The American Diabetes Association, The American Heart Association and the American Cancer Association recommend nutrient-rich legumes as a key food group for preventing disease and optimizing health. Legumes are rich in protein, fiber, minerals, vitamins and phytonutrients. They are low-fat, no cholesterol, low-glycemic-index foods. The University of Michigan Health System recommends one to three servings of beans and legumes a day.

George Mateljan, author of *The World's Healthiest Foods* and the founder of The Mateljan Foundation, says kidney beans are a very good source of cholesterol-lowering fiber, as are most other beans. In addition to lowering cholesterol, kidney beans' high fiber content prevents blood sugar levels from rising too rapidly after a meal, making these beans an especially good choice for individuals with diabetes, insulin resistance or hypoglycemia. (See http://www.whfoods.com)

Hardcore Health: Live Young!

WATER

We are made of water, we live on a planet made predominantly of water, therefore it seems obvious that we are meant to ingest a lot of water (a medical fact, as in the survival world absence of water kills you before absence of food).

I try to guzzle water all day long— the more the better. And you may not agree with this, but I am a big believer in tap water and exposure to the local germs, as long as you are not an infant and your municipal water system is tested for the really toxic content. Once you get to be a full-grown adult, I don't think a few germs can hurt you and they may help build up your immune system.

Whatever your source, drink a lot of water, especially before any physical activity or training session. We are running a factory in our body and water is the driving force. In keeping with the 80% super diet and 20% eat-whatever-you-want, the same goes for fluids. I try to drink only water, or light beer if I am going for a stimulant. The 20% of the time you can go wild and have sugar water (soda) or go all the way and have a milk shake and/or a shot of tequila or a glass of full octane beer.

A 2013 report in the *International Journal of Endocrinology* states that the barley and hops in beer make it a good source of the mineral silicon, important for bone formation and health. Even better, it's the type of silicon that is easy for your bones to absorb. (See https://www.aarp.org/health/healthy-living/info-2015/mens-health-tips.html)

One of the most reliable gauges of a person's health is how their waste system is working, volume and quality especially, but I gladly will not go into detail on this. Think about it: would you use a tiny amount and/or contaminated version of motor oil or coolant for your car? No way. Then why would you do it with the one model vehicle you are stuck with? Think of water as your body's motor oil.

Nutrition consultant, body building guru and author of *The Health Handbook*, Chris Aceto explains that the consensus in the bodybuilding community is that high water storage within muscles acts as an anabolic factor. This allows the muscles to maintain a positive nitrogen balance, which directly impacts muscle growth. Just like plants, our muscles need water to grow.

The International Sports Medicine Institute recommends: 1/2 ounce per pound of body weight if you're not active, that's ten 8-ounce glasses of water for the 160-pounder, and 2/3 ounce per pound if you're athletic (13-to-14 glasses per day at the same weight).

Make sure you drink water before and after you exercise. (See http://www.bodybuilding.com.)

POOP WATCH

Hardcore Health: Live Young!

Though I know it sounds disgusting and commonly is, it is critical to observe composition of your bowel movements (visually) as it is one of the best indicators of your health. Making poop should be a natural and easy process—if it is too hard or too soft that usually means there are problems in the factory we call our digestive system.

The worst thing you can see in your poop, of course, is blood and you should immediately seek out professional help. Other things that may shock you, especially the first time you see them, are likely harmless, e.g. corn niblets.

As in the efficiency of any factory, you need to make sure the pipes get fully cleaned out every day or you might have blockages or stoppages that might be detrimental to overall body (factory) performance. People always roll their eyes when I tell them I am a quasi-beanatarian in regard to the obvious reference to expelling rectal gas (farting)! Passing gas is actually a very healthy action that is one of the first signs of recovery after surgery. It indicates the factory is working properly. I must have built up a strong resistance (or at least my wife has) to my massive bean and cabbage daily consumption. Believe it or not, I don't pass gas that often and when I do, they don't seem to smell bad, (a reference to the elitist saying that he/she thinks "their shit doesn't smell")!

I believe your body gets used to digesting certain foods like beans and cabbage, handling them without fanfare—whereas a new initiate might have problems initially digesting some of the colon-blow or colon-cleanse food types. My suggestion is to stick with it (and provide your partner with a gas mask) until your system can handle these extremely healthy, yet potentially explosive foods!

According to Jonathan Isbit of *Nature's Platform*, nature has deliberately created obstacles to evacuation that can only be removed by squatting. In any other position, the colon defaults to "continence mode." This is why the conventional sitting position deprives the colon of support from the thighs and leaves the rectum choked by the puborectalis muscle. These obstacles make elimination difficult and incomplete.

Chronically incomplete evacuation, combined with the constant extraction of water, causes wastes to adhere to the colon wall. The passageway becomes increasingly constricted and the cells start to suffocate. Prolonged exposure to toxins will often trigger malignant mutations.

He goes on to explain how the kink where your sigmoid joins your rectum serves an important function in continence. It "applies the brakes" to the flow of peristalsis, reducing the pressure on your puborectalis muscle. According to Isbit's article, squatting gives many advantages. It helps prevent fecal stagnation, a prime factor in colon cancer, stops chronic straining that can cause hernias, is a non-invasive treatment for hemorrhoids, helps constipation by lifting the sigmoid colon and unlocks the kink at the entrance to the rectum. It also avoids pressure on the uterus for pregnant women. (See www.naturesplatform.com/health_benefits.html)

Dr. Mercola in a health article on bowel movements recommends checking the internet for devices on the marketplace like the Squatty Potty. This recent multi-million dollar invention seen on the TV series Shark Tank is a simple footstool type apparatus that fits around the stem of the toilet. With your feet, and therefore your knees, higher, your body assumes a more squatty position. (https://articles.mercola.com/sites/articles/archive/2012/.../toilet-squatting-position.aspx)

EXERCISE

Studies show that one of the greatest hidden health threats we all face is sitting too much. Prolonged sitting negatively affects hearth health, blood fats, blood sugar, blood pressure, hormone levels, bones, organs, liver, kidneys and pancreas.

Dr. James Levine, an endocrinologist and author of *Get Up! Why Your Chair is Killing You and What You Can do About It,* says at least two dozen chronic diseases and conditions are associated with excessive sitting. The human body is meant to be active all day and was never designed to be crammed into a chair where all of these cellular mechanisms get switched off.

What can you do about it? Try:
>   Take a five-minute walk for every thirty minutes sitting.
>   Stand at your workstation, while on the phone or while watching TV.
>   Lift weights or pedal a stationary bike while watching TV.
>   Take the stairs not the elevator.
>   Park far from your destination and walk.
>   Exercise!
>   Stretch regularly.

High and Low-Impact Sports

The smartest thing I ever did for my body was quitting high impact sports when I was 25 years old. It was an easy transition as I had just arrived in Hawaii, the Mecca of (low impact) world-class surfing and a marginal place for basketball, the land sport I loved. I was a gym rat growing up in Florida between ocean flat spells, which are excruciatingly long and common. The caliber of athleticism in Florida was unrivaled and I became a respected basketball player, even making the finals of a One-on-One contest at Florida State University where I played in front of 10,000 people.

Upon arriving in Hawaii, the waves and ocean were much more alluring. Many of my friends were experiencing serious knee/ankle/shoulder injuries from high-impact sports, thus making my decision to quit very easy.

Hardcore Health: Live Young!

Note that I define high-impact sports as any land sport where your full body weight is landing repeatedly and violently on the ground. This includes all land sports, as well as running.

It just makes way more sense to stop abusing your joints. If you don't believe that land sports are violent to your body, I encourage you to look up the slow motion video of the impact your knees or ankles take every time they hit the ground —quite shocking, literally and figuratively!

On the other hand, low-impact sports are equally as fun and can be performed for the rest of your life. If you add water, it gets even better as the weight of your body is reduced when submerged!

Here are the classic low-impact sports/activities that I highly recommend:

Walking
Biking
Swimming
Paddling.

There is no excuse for not being able to perform the first two, even if you do them at home using a treadmill and/or stationary bike.

As a primitive creature, I prefer to perform these tasks out in nature. The other key element for me is that I hate to exercise just to exercise, but rather prefer to work my daily low-impact activities into achieving required objectives via my required errands/chores/work breaks.

I perform the following three main low-impact activities to meet these requirements: Walk, Bike, Paddle/Swim/Dive. Note that these activities in combination are also an excellent way to cross-train (working all the different muscle groups) with the eye on the prize: paddling into big waves on the North Shore!

Any sport you enjoy will help improve physical health and mental well-being, a potential contribution to increased life-expectancy. In a 2011 NCBI study, older male golfers performed much better on several different tests of balance and physical confidence than men of the same age who did not golf. Walking the course had more benefits, of course, than riding in a golf cart. (https://www.ncbi.nlm.nih.gov/m/pubmed/21416145/)

To Train or Not to Train

Many athletes, young or not-so-young, often neglect training, as most people want to get right down to the fun part of performing the sport itself. One of my good friends in my twenties was a golf prodigy, the only problem was he hated practicing and only loved to play golf. He would play 18 holes a day, but never made the Tour. The professionals that ultimately make it on the Tour don't just play rounds of golf, they hit hundreds or thousands of the same shot to perfect each and every shot they might encounter during a round of golf.

Hardcore Health: Live Young!

I try to do the same for surfing. I train to surf and surf to train. Instead of just surfing whenever I can on whatever waves are available, I would rather do my 2-mile paddle/dive/swim event that is designed to prepare me for when the big waves roll into the North Shore. That way, when my leash snaps or my board breaks and I am one mile from shore and have to swim under twenty mountains of water in a row, I can relax (a little) knowing that I trained for that exact same situation all week leading up to that event. Everyone wants the glory of riding a big wave, however not that many people are willing to train for it. Fortunately for me, I have devised a training regimen that I really enjoy and that is so enthralling itself that I hardly realize that I am actually training and not just having fun!

Note that when the waves get big on the North Shore, a big misconception is that only young people are out there—it is actually just the opposite with more people in their 40's to 60's then people in their 20's. One reason is that waves like that take a lot of experience and 20 year olds just don't have it (yet). The other reason is, of course, lack of training—it's just not that sexy for most people to paddle for two miles at a clip without the reward of actually surfing. Big wave surfing can be summed up in four words: "board speed and ball weight." You need to propel your surfboard as fast as possible to get into the larger wave as early and as easy as possible, i.e., miles of paddle training, and you have to have the balls (guts) to look down from the top of a massive wall of water and say *I am going down the mountain and I am not going to die!*

Walking

I walk the dogs half a mile twice a day. This is an easy way to get a couple of good brisk walks under your belt. I highly recommend getting one or more dogs to force you to get into this habit. It also serves as a great mental break during your day or when you get home from work or after dinner as it is the only time you can stop and ponder nature without the neighbors calling the cops on the crazy guy lingering around staring into space. With dogs you have an excuse!

Just taking the dogs for a walk can change your whole attitude. First of all, they are so grateful to be going outside, and you should be too! For a while, we had three dogs and I prided myself on being able to walk all three at once. It was a moving carnival, especially since the trio consisted of a lab, a rottweiler, and a poodle type of dog someone gave my wife.

One of the basic challenges was cleaning up the dog poop of one dog while keeping the other two constrained. Not only did I have to keep the one dog in the process from being disturbed, as I hold pooping in high regard as one of the required bodily functions, but I also had to keep the other dogs from stepping in the newly minted load, or worse yet, dragging me through it. It was like juggling or spinning plates. Once in while I would get lucky and have all three of them poop at the same time like a choreographed orchestra performance—the trifecta!

Another walking technique is to purposely park your car in the furthest spot in any parking lot and briskly walk in and out of stores as required. I personally have a three mile and 50 lb. rule. If the errand I need to run is within three miles of my house/office and involves carrying weights of 50 lbs. or less, than it falls into the Bike category.

Some of the benefits of exercise come directly from its ability to reduce insulin resistance, reduce inflammation, and stimulate the release of growth factors—chemicals in the brain that affect the health of brain cells, the growth of new blood vessels in the brain, and even the abundance and survival of new brain cells. (https://www.ncbi.nlm.nih.gov/pmc/articles/PMC3782965/)

Walking leads to more creative thinking, according to a recent study from researchers at Stanford University. Fans of the walk and talk include Facebook chief Mark Zuckerberg, Twitter co-founder Jack Dorsey and Barack Obama. Facebook recently put in a half-mile loop on the roof of its new headquarters in Menlo Park, California and LinkedIn workers stroll and talk on the bike path at the company's Mountain View,

California, headquarters. The walk and talks have obvious benefits. Desk-bound office workers can all use a bit more exercise. Sitting too much is killing us. Walking also helps break down formalities and fosters camaraderie between colleagues.

Biking

My mountain bike has straight across handle bars, a narrow plastic basket in the back, and two cloth shopping bags that can be hung on each side of the handle bars for big loads. Since a lot of my work requires that I do not sustain brain damage, I wear a helmet at all times. The helmet also has the advantage of blocking the sun from my head and the ladies think I am some hot looking young dude—until I take my helmet off and they see my age wrinkles/sun tattoos. I earned those tattoos anyway so it is quite amusing, at least to me!

The other great advantage of biking is the lack of problems with parking and traffic. There is no better feeling than passing a cue of cars waiting at a light or in a parking lot as the wind flies through my hair. On the green side, there is also the bonus of saving energy and it's nice to know I have unlimited miles per gallon while I pedal away.

For errands that are further than three miles, I commonly will throw the bike in the trunk of the car and park within a few miles of the destination (e.g., downtown) and cruise in using the same techniques. The helmet is even more critical on those trips as town traffic has a higher degree of risk and difficulty.

At the moment, scientists don't completely understand the exact mechanisms, but they know that physical activity like cycling boosts the production of feel-good chemicals such as serotonin and dopamine. J. David Glass, PhD, a brain-chemistry researcher at Kent State University in Kent, Ohio, reports that lab rats get a 100% to 200% increase in serotonin levels when running on their wheels.

Paddle/Dive/Swim

As an aging big wave surfer, everything I do physically is centered around keeping me in the game on the North Shore for as long as possible and also, more importantly, preventing me from dying in the deadly large surf and associated currents.

Before the massive explosion of stand-up paddle boarding—including my invention of the inflatable paddleboard—traditional paddle boarding consisted of lying down on a board and paddling in the prone position, the same exact motion of paddling for surfing purposes. I have a 25+ year old traditional paddleboard that is half water-logged that I paddle two miles a day. I like the added weight of the massive/heavy board as when I am on my real surfboards they feel light and easy to paddle!

A few years ago, I almost drowned on a big North Shore day. A huge set of waves came in that were about 40 feet high on their faces. My 12-foot North Shore "gun" (pointy) surfboard and my 20-foot leash were dragged like toys and I became a rag doll. The leash stretched to about 40 feet long and kept me right in the impact zone where the waves were breaking. I had to take one breath and dive down under about 12 feet of whitewater, then come up for air to do the same thing for about twenty waves in a row. When I finally got to the beach, and kissed the sand, I was tired for a week!

As a scientist/inventor, I analyzed the situation over and over in my head and simply came to the conclusion that I need to practice for that exact situation by simulating it every day, thus leading to what is now my daily lunchtime (pre-meal) paddle break:

Loin Cloth Water—Ape Paddle Event
Equipment required:
1 loin cloth (swimwear) with pocket
Polarized sunglasses with small fishing float tied to them
Sunscreen (or long sleeve UV inhibitor rash guard)
Paint roller for applying sunscreen to my back
12-foot prone paddleboard
25-foot piece of line

After lubing up, perform a series of leg/arm/shoulder stretches, followed by twelve "get-ups." A "get-up" consists of lying flat on the ground

Hardcore Health: Live Young!

and then in one smooth motion jumping to your feet to simulate standing up on a surfboard as you drop into a wave. This is an incredible exercise that is perfectly suited for an aging surfer as our flexibility and reflexes begin to lag.

Get into water and paddle for one mile or twenty minutes. Work on your paddle technique and breathing. The nice thing about the traditional paddleboard is that they glide so efficiently through the water that it feels like a 6-inch wave is always pushing you. I like to get a little warmed up after a few minutes and then jump off the board and get completely wet and then keep paddling. Depending on the climate you are in, you can alter the frequency and degree in which you want to get wet.

After one mile/twenty minutes, I jump off the board into the water and tie the 25-foot string around the board in front of the fin and flip the board over to tow the board along as I dive/swim. A mistake I made early on was keeping the bottom of my board white, making it resemble a whitecap, resulting in literally being run over by a boat. Fortunately, Louie Zamperini reminded me never to be tied to anything when you are in the water and that it is better to wrap lines to you. My 25-foot string was wrapped around my hand while I was in the water and I therefore was able to get rid of the board (by getting the rope off my hand and thus untangling myself from the board) and dive down twenty feet underwater and watch the powerboat run over my board and drag it for 1,000 yards.

I lived through that near-death experience and now my board is painted bright orange on the bottom! I should have known this lesson, as my See/Rescue Streamer invention is based on linear orange targets! It would be a terrible story if the inventor of a high visibility signaling device was run over because no one could see him!

Ultra fit surfer Laird Hamilton in a *Men's Journal* Aug 15, 2013 interview says that like swimming, paddle boarding is an all-body workout. It strengthens your core and stabilization system, requiring your connective tissue to generate power through your hands and out your feet. But more than just the physical rewards, paddle boarding restores your balance and calms your spirit.

One-Breath Free Dives

Once the board is flipped over and you have the string tied to it and wrapped to your hand, proceed to perform twenty one-breath free dives in a row to simulate that North Shore near-death experience. From my free diving experience, I learned the free dive/snorkeling technique of curling your legs up into a crouch as you rotate downward to propel yourself underwater. It is actually quite easy and natural once you get the hang of it. I dive down ten feet deep and then come up for one breath of air and repeat for twenty times in a row (one breath only between free dives) to simulate that experience of getting caught by twenty waves in a row. (Note: This is not hyperventilating at all but rather mellowing out or slowing down your breathing (it's like Yoga underwater—Woga!)

One of my favorite things in the world is being submerged and weightless in the ocean. This routine fulfills this desire and at the same time provides an incredible training exercise to give me even more confidence under pressure during big North Shore waves. I also figured out that, when I come up from the twelve feet depth, I can twist my body to the left or right or backwards, thereby working my mid-section/core. I used to do 100 sit ups every night. I haven't done one sit up in seven years since I started doing this and my stomach/core is in better shape than ever. In essence, I am performing underwater yoga moves with the water providing a gravitational relief and making it much easier to flex my body—as opposed to the complete agony of doing a traditional sub-aerial sit up!

Avoid Ear Infections

On the subject of swimming and diving, for a while I had trouble with ear infections. A trick I learned many moons ago from our kids' pediatrician is the simple procedure of mixing rubbing alcohol and white vinegar to make your own ear drops to prevent ear infections.

Note that you should use standard rubbing alcohol, but could use other types in a pinch. During one of my surf trips deep into mainland Mexico, I used tequila! As for vinegar, make sure you use white vinegar and not something like balsamic vinegar, unless you want ants and cockroaches having a fiesta in your ear.

Simply mix the alcohol and vinegar in 50/50 proportions and place in a generic eye-dropper or other dispenser. I presently use a plastic ketchup dispenser in my bathroom since the drug stores don't like selling you empty dispenser bottles as it cuts into their sales of over the counter medicine. After each time you get wet—shower, surfing, rain shower, etc. —simply shake your mixture bottle and place several drops in each ear. I haven't had an earache in 25+ years and I used to get them all the time! The only downfall is your partner might have to get used to the slight vinegar smell, especially when it drips out of your ear while you are kissing.(Note to self: put in ears after and not before an amorous activity.)

Rough Water Swim

Following the one-breath free dives, I like to swim for several hundred yards to simulate the situation where my leash breaks and I have to swim to the beach and/or find my board that has drifted away. Swimming is also a fantastic overall exercise that contributes to my overall comfort in big North

Hardcore Health: Live Young!

Shore surf, as I know in the worst case scenario, I can always swim if I have to.

Another thing unique to diving and swimming is that they are pure loin cloth activities, i.e., no swim aids of any kind are used, no fins, no mask, no snorkel to serve as crutches. It's just you and the ocean (or lake or pool).

At the World Aquatic Health Conference Sept, 2008, Dr. Steven Blair was asked if swimming reduced the risk of dying. His answer was an enthusiastic yes. Dr. Blair's study, over the course of 32 years, followed 40,000 men, ranging from 20 to 90 years old and discovered that those who swam had a 50% lower death rate than runners, walkers or men who got no exercise.
(https://www.nspf.org/sites/default/files/sitefinity/Files/Blair_May09_WaterShapes.pdf)

In 2009, a Belgian review article in *Clinical Rehabilitation* found sufficient evidence to conclude that aquatic exercise is a safe and effective way to relieve chronic low-back pain. And a 2006 Swedish study found that water exercise reduced the incidence of back pain in pregnant women. Working out in water reduces the stress on the spine, promotes muscle relaxation and improves joint flexibility.
(https://www.ncbi.nlm.nih.gov/pubmed/16881990)

A Jun, 2014 study showed that aquatic exercise, using the water's buoyancy, helps decrease body fat while maintaining superior mobility.

Swimming also improves physical strength, endurance, and flexibility, and is a great workout because you need to move your whole body against the resistance of the water. It keeps your heart rate up but takes some of the impact stress off your body. (https://www.ncbi.nlm.nih.gov/pmc/articles/PMC4106774/)

Paddle/Belly Ride

The final one mile/twenty minutes of this workout consists of paddling back in and catching one wave on the way back to shore, thus making it an official "surf" session. As traditional paddleboards are too narrow and light to stand up on, you must ride the waves lying down on your belly. A belly ride is quite a challenge/workout as you have to slide back on the board so the nose doesn't sink and flip you over. You also can drag your arms or legs as needed to slow down and/or change direction.

Usually, I am laughing all the way as this replicates my first experiences riding waves when I was a little grom on an inflatable raft. Also, believe it or not, I have had some of the longest waves of my life on my belly as the smallest of waves can continue to push you along. It's also a nice reward after your free dive/rough water swim.

(The ultimate goal when you approach 100-years-of-age as a surfer is to join the "Belly Leash Club"—that is when your ankles are too brittle to wear a surf leash around them and instead you wear the leash around your belly—a goal that was inspired by the must-see movie *Surfing For Life* featuring 90-year-old surfers still surfing and having a ball!)

Finally, after I get to shore, I reward myself with my Push Button Super Fuel Feast. There is nothing like eating a great meal that you feel you've earned. If people would match their food intake to the energy they exerted prior to eating it, they would be in much better shape (i.e. "do more, eat less" and not the other way around)! Most humans, as they age, do the exact opposite and eat more and do less! Perhaps only let yourself eat after you have completed some physical exercise/exertion and match the proportions—a one block walk gets a tiny meal and a five mile walk gets the feast!

My ocean paddling/dive/swim regimen is training for my ultimate passion of big wave surfing. Everyone needs to find their own passion and balance the training aspect with the ultimate event itself. If you love to hike up mountains, you can't do it every day, however you can train every day for the once a week or month you get to actually scale a peak. You need to find your own physical passion. It doesn't even have to be in nature, however I believe that adds another dimension to it.

I also highly recommend choosing something that you can do alone, both the training and execution of the actual event. Self-reliance (thanks Emerson and Thoreau) is a key theme for me as it removes the hassle of relying on other people to achieve your objectives. Of course, you can do group events and those can be fun, however if you design a program that you can do alone and at anytime you will be much more likely to keep it going for the long term. In keeping with the low impact theme, I would look at options that include water since those are the ultimate in low impact, especially if you are submerged where the weight of your body is reduced, and that is a nice bonus!

Physical Maintenance

It's fairly easy to be a great physical specimen when you are in your 20's, but keeping it up in your 50's and beyond is another story. The diet and exercise regime described above is a great baseline to keep you in your optimum shape.

Just as ample water is the key for your diet, I believe it is the key for your external body/skin appearance too. I think it is no secret how the human body feels when it is submerged in a hot bath or a cool, clean ocean. All of your pores seem to explode and breathe when you are wet. If something feels that good, it makes sense that you should try to recreate that state as often as possible throughout your life. Many fancy skin treatments revolve around some liquid or another. Therefore, stay wet as often as possible, both internally and externally.

Hardcore Health: Live Young!

Staying Fit in the City

If you happen to live in a city or suburb with no access to the ocean or mountains, you will just have to be more creative. Envision the streets and sidewalks as a type of nature or mountain (cave) trail.

The first and easiest thing to do is my preferred mode for all exercise—don't make it exercise, make it part of your normal daily routine. An energetic/large dog will need to be walked a few times a day. Walking at a brisk pace is one of the best workouts of all. You don't need any equipment and you can even do it without dogs, however dogs make it much easier to be more creative on your route and the time you spend admiring little nooks and crannies of your city/mountain. Dogs give you a good front to meander around and they force you to pick up the pace.

Walking can also be incorporated into your daily required routine. The three mile/50 pound rule I use for biking can be lowered to two mile/25 pounds whereby if your errand (post office/store/bank) is that close to your house or office, then it's a walking trip, or biking if you prefer. You can even go old-school and bring a fold-up rolling cart—like the elderly ladies; however, you can rock it if you are really hardcore!

Hardcore walking also applies to how you interact with your car. Always park in the furthest spot in any parking lot. It's counterintuitive, but it is really smarter. Aside from the exercise and fresh air before you go into a land structure, you don't sit and waste gas and time looking for parking spots that make you lazier with a shorter walk. Parking far away is a different mindset, but once you try it, you might like it. The other nice thing about this technique is that if you live in a remote area and the 2 mile/25 pound rule does not apply, you can compensate for that by conducting your errands from a remote parking spot.

    The other key is to try and walk briskly on your way to and from the land structure and within the structure itself. For the really hardcore, you can travel with your bike in your car trunk and park a few miles away from any remote location/meeting site. Forced long walks also apply to city parking where you can park on the top or bottom of the structure and use the stairs, and of course use the stairs whenever possible in all buildings once you get in. One obvious side benefit of this is you have no chance of getting stuck in an elevator.

    If you live somewhere with severe weather, you can always buy one or both of the best pieces of old school home workout equipment: stationary bike and/or treadmill. Once again the theme is low-impact (easy on the knees/joints/backs) biking or walking. I also like to exercise the same muscles as I use for longer versions—just as the lay-down paddleboard prepares you for the same physical

Hardcore Health: Live Young!

motion as surfing, exercise bikes/treadmills train your muscles for long bike rides and long walks. You can also multi-task when you are on stationary exercise equipment, however be careful not to get hurt, especially on the treadmill. My family members have used this multi-tracking trick for years, reading books and now even watching movies on the stationary equipment, taking your mind off the physical exertion and making the time go fast!

As in the nature exercising described earlier, try to reward yourself with a meal after each city/suburb exercise event, e.g., walk to your meals, eat after you walk the dogs, or run, bike or walk your errands. By combining a physical exertion that becomes your routine with your daily health meals, you will see immediate results on your overall health and even energy level.

Explore Google for free fitness programs and also check in with your local Parks and Recreation Department. Minnesota, for example, offers a summer-long fitness series in nine city parks (stpaul.gov/fitnessintheparks). Non profits like the November Project offer free outdoor workouts in 19 cities (november-project.com). New York's Shape Up NYC Program has free kickboxing and circuit-training classes (nycgovparks.org). The Museum of Science at the University of Chicago offers a community fitness program where you can join fitness walks inside of the world's most famous museums 7.30 am to 9 am on Monday, Wednesday and Friday

Check Meetup and Goiety for like-minded groups and social Apps like WeGoDo and Sesh that connect those looking for running, cycling, climbing or skiing buddies.

Cities offering indoor bike paths include Ray's in Cleveland, Wheel Mill in Pittsburgh and Sranx in Syracuse, NY. Mega Cavern is a seven-acre park beneath Louisville, KY with impressive dirt tracks. Los Angeles CA has Sender One, a cool climbing gym and Twin Cities has Midwest Climbing Academy and a chain of climbing gyms.

Want to stretch and contort as you scale a fiendishly designed route to attain the summit? Dogpatch Boulders, in San Francisco, is the largest bouldering gym in the country and Planet Granite has three challenging bouldering gyms in the Bay area and one in Portland, Oregon. Hangar 18 Indoor Climbing Gyms in Southern California offers indoor climbing with over 55,000ft of textured climbing terrain, world-class bouldering, and massive lead caves featuring routes up to 70ft long.

Water parks like Schlitterbahn Water Parks in Texas and FlowRider at Planet Hollywood Resort, Las Vegas, offer mountains of water to surf even though you are miles away from the ocean.

YOUR SKIN AND NON-SURGICAL SOLUTIONS TO MAKE YOU LOOK YOUTHFUL

Jennifer Armstrong MS, MD, Advanced Skincare Surgery and Medcenter, Newport Beach CA.

Skin is your largest organ. It accounts for about 15% of your body weight. Your skin protects your vital organs and aids temperature regulation. But that is not all. Skin can be aesthetically pleasing as well as a window to disease in the body. The average person has about 300 million skin cells. Skin is made of the epidermis (outer layer), dermis (where collagen, sweat glands, and hair follicles live) and the subcutaneous fat layer which consists of fat and larger vessels and nerves.

The cell types of the epidermis are many, but keratinocytes and melanocytes are the most known. Melanocytes release melanin containing melanosomes, which give us freckles and a sun tan. They also give rise to melanoma, the deadliest of skin cancers. In the dermal layer, a single square inch of skin has up to 300 sweat glands. Your skin constantly sheds, renewing itself every 28 days. A person sheds nearly 9 lbs. of dead skin cells per year! Your skin is its thickest on your feet, about 1.4mm, and thinnest on your delicate eyelids, about 0.2mm.

Protect Your Skin

The best thing you can do for your skin is to protect it, avoiding the sun from 10am – 2pm. If you are out enjoying life, always protect with a sun block not a sunscreen. Zinc will block the radiation effects of the sun. THINK ZINC. Titanium Dioxide works well too.

For some unknown reason, people tend to think they only need sunscreen when it is sunny out. Well, actually you need it every day the sun rises. So use it daily.

If your skin is damaged as a child, you will see it when you are an adult. The body is constantly trying to mend the DNA of the damaged cells in your youth but over time it will present itself as actinic keratosis or a skin cancer.

Get That Glow

There are many lasers and topical creams you can use to make your skin glow. If you would like to do inexpensive home versions that work, here are a few tricks: After eating a delicious papaya, lay the papaya skin on your face. Due to the presence of Papain, papaya is an excellent exfoliant. Papain dissolves dead skin cells and thus aids in skin exfoliation. Leave on for 10min and then rinse your face. It will feel soft and smooth.

Try growing aloe and applying it (or any moisturizer) within 5 minutes after showering. This locks in moisture.

Hardcore Health: Live Young!

Reduce Skin Damage Caused By UV Rays

If you are an active person and often out in the sun, carrots will reduce skin damage caused by UV rays. Carotenoids in carrots fight against free radicals which age us by decreasing elasticity and cause cancer through oxidation. So what do you need? Anti-oxidants. Carrots have high amounts of Vitamin A which is a good antioxidant and fights free radicals.

Carrots can be applied topically, too. Prepare or buy a cup of carrot juice, dip some cotton into carrot juice and wipe onto the face and neck. Rinse with cold water after 5 minutes. What you put into your body also matters, not just topical applications.

Prevent Aging

Want to prevent aging? Eat blueberries. Blueberries have high amounts of antioxidants that combat free radicals.

Wash your face every night, moisturize and combat damage with antioxidants and protect your skin with zinc. That's it!

Non-surgical Solutions to Make You Look Youthful

In general using a Retin A type product will help increase skin cell turnover, will help improve and prevent fine lines and wrinkles and will give your skin a nice glow. The problem is that these medications require a prescription. You can find skincare products that contain a derivative of Retin A (called retinol) that is also helpful. Lastly, you will want to wear sunblock daily because sun exposure is aging in and of itself.

Fraxel Laser Skin Resurfacing
Fraxel Laser skin resurfacing is an effective treatment for improving the tone and texture of your skin. The benefits include smoother, fresher looking skin, reduced wrinkles, reduced pore size, and improved skin tone. Fraxel Light energy stimulates collagen and the effects are immediate and long lasting. Three to five sessions four to five weeks apart work well. Always go to a dermatologist or plastic surgeon. All medical procedures have risks.

Restoring Volume To Your Face
If you want something non surgical, then I suggest you use Botox for the lines in the upper face, and fillers to address volume loss to the lower face. Voluma helps restore lost volume, and then other hyaluronic acid fillers work for the area around your mouth. Sculptra would also be an option to help regain some lost volume.

Soften Wrinkles and Crows Feet Under The Eyes
Hollowness under the eyes in the tear trough area can be helped by the use of fillers. The fine

lines and crepey skin under the eyes can also be helped with a combination of Botox and fillers. Make sure you go to someone who performs a lot of tear trough injections.

In general, this area is best treated as a combination therapy. If you are wanting to avoid a surgical procedure, then laser resurfacing, micro needling with PRP and/or stem cells or fillers all work great in this area. Botox works very well for crows feet correction around the eyes.

Soften Lines Around Lips

Typically a filler would help to soften lines around the lips. You can also do some Botox for the vertical lip lines above your lip.

Vertical lip lines can be treated in several different ways, often requiring multiple different treatment modalities. Small amounts of Botox to stop the pursing lip movement, hyaluronic acid fillers like Volbella to fill in the lines, fractional CO_2 laser resurfacing, and also micro needling with PRP treatments are all viable options for these pesky lines. Stopping smoking should also be a must if you are serious about stopping these lines.

Stimulate Collagen

As the years pass, the skin's deepest layer stops producing collagen at the rate it did in the past and appearance suffers. Once-youthful firm skin begins to wrinkle, sag, and droop as the strength and quality of collagen lessens. Ultherapy creates an environment that stimulates the body to regenerate and produce more of this critical element of firm skin. As it is your own collagen, the results can be dramatic and natural.

Ultherapy is FDA approved to treat face and neck skin laxity, brow lifting, chest skin revitalization, under chin looseness, and facial skin rejuvenation. Ultherapy treatment is an alternative to facelift surgery and appropriate for those who are living with the earlier stages of aging skin. An Ultherapy treatment doesn't replace a facelift procedure, but can be an excellent alternative, particularly for patients who don't want to undergo a surgical procedure. For older patients who have extensive wrinkling, sagging, and drooping, Ultherapy can be used as an added procedure to prolong the results of surgery. Most patients need only one treatment, but every person is different, living with varying degrees of skin laxity and the degree to which their skin responds. Always go to a board-certified dermatologist or plastic surgeon. All medical procedures have risks.

Botox Neck lift

Botox can also be used to temporarily improve the appearance of the neck by relaxing the platysmal bands. This treatment works by reducing the activity of these muscles. The procedure, also known as Botox Neck Lift, is quick and has minimal downtime.

Solutions for Sun Damage On Chest

Sun damage on the chest is a very common concern, as it is an area that receives a large amount of sun exposure and thus sun damage. The treatment options vary depending on your ethnic background, skin type, and level of sun damage. One method is IPL, or Intense Pulsed Light, which can be an effective treatment for some patients. This procedure is best performed in months where you have little or no sun exposure. There are also a variety of other treatments which include a variety of laser treatments or topical medications.

Venus Versa IPL targets the spots which will darken and then disappear.

Solutions For Acne and Oily Skin

If your skin is sensitive and oily and you have problems with acne, I would highly recommend a topical treatment known as a retinoid. There are many different types of retinoids available, some are over the counter formulations like Retinol or Adapalene, but there are also prescription strength medications such as Retin A. They can take up to 90 days to be effective. Different strengths work for different individuals so it can take some time to find the exact regimen that works with your skin type.

Solutions For Large Pores, Skin Tone and Texture

A fractional resurfacing treatment helps with pore size, skin tone & texture. There are many different treatments on the market and every patient's specific needs are different.

HAIR
Washing

As a young lad, I remember meeting my grandfather briefly and he had this incredible long, thick white hair. Perhaps he was a little senile, but when I asked him how he had such a massive pile of hair when most people his age were thinning or balding, he told me the secret is to never wash your hair. I think he was referring to the chemicals in the soap or shampoo, but I never received confirmation on that theory. Nevertheless, how many bald homeless people have you ever seen? Not many, as they mostly seem to have thick, albeit matted and often nasty hair. Perhaps there is something to that!

Fast forward to my present senior citizen status age and I still have hair—it's definitely thinner in spots, but I definitely have it. It is likely genetic, but I don't expose it to the harsh chemicals in shampoo and conditioners and like to think that has helped. By the way, if you really want to scare yourself, read the ingredients label on a shampoo bottle and then think about pouring those chemicals into your head's hot-water-induced, wide-open pores.

My strategy is to keep your hair clean by rinsing with clean cool ocean water and hot clean shower water, with a once a week shampoo.

For men, one other tip on hair and it's probably a placebo, is to ingest a saw palmetto vitamin every day. I read that saw palmetto is good for your hair, although it is hard to prove scientifically. It turns out saw palmetto is also supposed to be good for your prostate health—so right there it is a double bonus for men, as you avoid doctors and hospitals as much as possible, not to mention keeping your sensitive private parts away from cold probing metal instruments—unless of course you're into that.

James A. Duke, Ph.D., leading authority on healing herbs and author of *The Green Pharmacy,* explains that saw palmetto may indeed promote hair growth since it inhibits conversion of testosterone to dihydrotestosterone (DHT) not unlike Propecia, the FDA approved drug. The recommended dose is 160 mg of an extract standardized to 85-95% total fatty acids twice daily.

New Ways to Fight Baldness

Recent research shows that male sex hormones, most notably DHT, play a significant role in male pattern baldness and even in some female hair loss. Hair follicles on the front and crown of the head have receptors for DHT while the hair follicles on the sides and back of the head do not. This accounts for the common patterns of hair loss which starts with a receding hairline at the front and a thinning of the hair at the crown of the head. (https://www.ncbi.nlm.nih.gov/pubmed/28396101)

  Research in December 2016 suggested minoxidil, finasteride, and low-level laser light therapy are effective for promoting hair growth in men with androgenetic alopecia and that minoxidil is effective in women with androgenetic alopecia. (https://www.ncbi.nlm.nih.gov/pubmed/28396101.) Hairmax Laser Comb is FDA approved.

  Studies show that most men experiencing hair loss can take a daily supplement of saw palmetto and beta sitosterol to stop their hair loss and allow for renewed growth. The combination of saw palmetto and beta sitosterol inhibit both forms of 5-alpha-reductase. Since these phytosterols are chemically similar to testosterone, they bind to and block 5-alpha-reductase from converting testosterone to DHT, the rogue hair-loss inducing hormone.

  A 24 week study of pumpkin oil supplements in 2014 showed a positive anabolic effect on hair growth and that this is due to the possible effects of 5-reductase inhibition in patients with mild to moderate male pattern hair loss. (https://www.ncbi.nlm.nih.gov/pmc/articles/PMC4017725/ lkementshttps://)

DHT can be blocked topically at the hair follicle. There are a variety of products that will do this from natural products that use saw palmetto, beta sitosterol, and various fatty acids. There are foam based and liquid based solutions.

Decreased blood flow and poor circulation to the roots can be a contributor of hair loss. Daily scalp and neck massages can help.

A team of German researchers found that topical applications of a caffeine lotion helps block the damaging effects of DHT on hair follicles and stimulates the growth of new hair. Researchers published their findings in the January 2007 issue of the *International Journal of Dermatology*. concluding that caffeine is a stimulator of human hair growth. There are shampoos containing caffeine such as Alpecin Caffeine Shampoo. (http://www.livestrong.com/article/550821-caffeine-dht/)

Latisse, the drug that thickens lashes might help your scalp. Check if your doctor will prescribe Latisse off-label to regrow hair.

On their very informative Hair Loss Review website, Berkeley Research Institute mentions supplement Hairomega for the quality of ingredients that have been proven to block DHT and provide hair follicles with the nutrients needed. For best topical solution, the Institute mentions Revivogen for the all-natural formulation ingredients, containing both DHT-blockers and growth

promoters.
(http://www.thehairlossreview.com/treatment_reviews.html)

TEETH

Shiny white teeth set in non-receding gums shout health and youth. They could shout wealth, too, as fixing teeth is expensive. Be that as it may, teeth are enormously important and losing them definitely proves that. Healthy gums are also important for your health.

Teeth can and will get worse, so take care of them. Not replacing missing teeth is a bad idea and will eventually affect the position of remaining teeth.

Obvious care for teeth is just what your mom or dentist probably told you:

Brush twice a day, from gums to the tip of your teeth.

Floss twice a day.

Cut back on sugar and sugary products, as these feed bacteria.

Cut back on food and drinks like coffee that will stain your teeth. Difficult, I know. Rinsing with water after drinking coffee or red wine helps. Fortunately porcelain veneers and crowns are highly stain resistant.

I am not a big fan of using anything artificial, either ingesting it or via some medical procedure. There is one simple breakthrough that enables you to feel semi-youthful as you grow long in the tooth—teeth whitening! I don't consider this fake as the hydrogen peroxide that is the base material is actually just cleaning your teeth of the stains accumulated over the years. (Use the 3% solution that says to use as a rinse or gargle). There is nothing like a good whitish smile to make you feel better in the morning as you look at yourself in the mirror. One caution I would suggest is to avoid the abrasive whitening products that keep wearing down your enamel and stick to the peroxide products that just chemically remove the stains, not the enamel. Note that its important to check the strength of the hydrogen peroxide and to limit the amount of time in which the product is used. Ask your dentist before rinsing with 3% hydrogen peroxide or a commercial peroxide product.

    Dr. Becky Ransey, holistic dentist, praises the benefits of 3% hydrogen peroxide. Dr. Ransey and her husband have been working in the medical field for over 36 years and recommend taking one capful (the little white cap that comes with the bottle), holding the hydrogen peroxide in your mouth for ten minutes daily, then spitting it out. She says you'll have no more canker sores and your teeth will be whiter without expensive plastic tapes and pastes. Let your toothbrushes soak in a cup of peroxide to keep them free of germs.

SUPPLEMENTS

Avoid the color white in food and avoid the color white in medicine, i.e., processed pharmaceutical pills. Keep all medicine you intake to an absolute minimum. Many people seem to live ingesting pills to solve problems across the board. Note that I am a total believer in Western medicine, just only as a last resort when you are really sick!

I do believe in vitamins, even though you should get most of your vitamins from your extremely healthy diet. The following vitamins are my base units that seem to help or at least help me think I am doing something good besides making my urine very expensive (absorption of pills where needed is suspect). I figure they can't hurt and they might help:

- Glucosamine with MSM (Joints/Ligaments for an aging athlete)
- Glucosamine with Chondroitin (Joints/Ligaments for an aging athlete)
- Calcium citrate (Bones)
- Fish oil (Brain)
- Saw palmetto (Prostate/Hair)
- Daily multiple vitamin (Overall)

The good stuff I get directly from my diet includes separate ingestion of cinnamon, ginger, turmeric, astaxanthin (found in salmon), flax seeds, chia seeds, hemp seeds, and of course blueberries. I know those are good for you as they were not made by a guy in a white coat (and they are not processed to the color white).

Hardcore Health: Live Young!

Astaxanthin, the natural compound that makes salmon, crabs, lobsters, shrimp and flamingos pink or red, has unique anti-aging potential. Reports highlight that astaxanthin is not an ordinary antioxidant by any stretch of the imagination. Its "clinical success extends beyond protection against oxidative stress and inflammation, to demonstrable promise for slowing age-related functional decline." Research continues at present and a first generation supplement is sold as ZanthoSyn.

There is one chemical I do ingest, as needed—Advil/Ibuprofen. I use it when I am injured to bring the swelling down so my body can heal. I know this works for me and I only take as many pills as directed. A few times in my life, I ramped up to a prescribed heavy duty anti-inflammatory, however that was when I was at my wits end and was approaching the prospect of shoulder surgery. It worked and I avoided surgery as my body was able to heal itself (see Rehab section below). As a rule though, I try to always go natural and avoid the chemicals, so I go with turmeric and Bio-Astin as my first two anti-inflammatory choices before I escalate to Advil/Ibuprofen or, if absolutely necessary, the prescription type.

In regard to emergency medicine, my go-to primitive solution for cuts or scrapes, coral reef or other, is gentian violet. This stuff has been around for 50+ years, but you can't find it too easily. It is purple-colored liquid that dries within five minutes of application and believe it or not is waterproof—the ultimate solution for a surfer that needs to get right back in the water without risking serious infections (critical if you are on a surf trip deep in a developing country).

I am convinced there is a conspiracy by the bandage and anti-biotic companies to prevent this stuff from getting on the shelf. It only costs a few bucks for a vial and it lasts for years—obviously not a very profitable business model. The one application I have heard it is still used for is for bull castration—where one swipe does the trick (who wants to go back for a second swipe)! Gentian Violet does have two minor problems: the purple stain it leaves on anything it touches and the shocking look you get from the general public when they look at a cut you have treated as the purple makes it look like a gnarly gunshot wound! I do have one rule regarding the purple stuff—never put it on your face—people will call the cops!

More old world primitive medical solutions can be found in the excellent reference book, *The Green Pharmacy*.

Karen Farid, DNP, CNS/CWON says European, Eastern European, Asian, Middle Eastern, and African/North African (Egypt, Morocco, Algiers) civilizations discovered gentian violet not only was a great dye, but it also had amazing abilities to eradicate skin (umbilical cord) and mucous membrane infections as well as promote wound healing.

    Pediatric practitioners were ahead of the rest of the medical/surgical community when they treated and eliminated cases of thrush (candida) infections of the mouth, even in nursing infants, who were exposed to candida infections of their mother's nipples. For decades, this has successfully treated lower extremity wounds, especially on elderly patients, and augmented the healing of pressure ulcers and abdominal wounds by applying gentian violet 1% solution to the wound edges to treat maceration and prevent migration of skin organisms into the wound. Gentian Violet is extremely well-tolerated (not a single sensitivity reaction), readily available, and inexpensive as an over-the-counter product in local pharmacies. Gentian Violet doesn't sting and can also be used on animals. From: Farid KJ, Kelly K, Roshin S. Gentian violet 1% solution in the treatment of wounds in the geriatric patient: a retrospective study. (Geriatr Nurs. 2011;32(2):85–95.)

MILD SEMI-NATURAL STIMULANTS

    As in the case of food and medicine, avoid the color white when considering recreational stimulants to relax, i.e. have a glass of wine or a beer instead of Valium or any other white chemical drug.

In moderation, I believe it is very useful to relax with a mild stimulant like beer or wine, especially if you combine it with a social or nature-based activity. Enjoy the slight stimulation enhanced by your friends and/or the environment. Down time is important in all aspects of life to not only recharge your batteries, but also to take a break from your daily grind. If I am in the midst of a major challenge, whether it is related to work or my personal life, I find it extremely useful to escape into nature and reset my mind. Some of my best work and creations come from my periods away from land and other humans, during my paddles.

Also, after a night of enjoying mild stimulants with friends—and laughing, another important ingredient—I commonly will wake up the next morning with a slightly new perspective on challenges that may have been hampering me the day before. It's almost like a reset button. I, of course, don't mean over-indulgence and losing consciousness, just a slight stimulant and laughter—a powerful combination!

A 2010 study from Johns Hopkins University suggests that red wine can diminish brain damage caused by stroke by as much as 40 percent. And recent research showed that grape-seed procyanidins, found in red wine, helps reduce arterial clogging, resulting in lower blood-cholesterol levels and a reduction in deaths from heart disease.

Hardcore Health: Live Young!

(https://www.hopkinsmedicine.org/news/media/releases/How_Red_Wine_May_Shield_Brain_From_Stroke_Damage)

The American Medical Association recommends men drink no more than two glasses of wine (10 ounces) a day and women one glass (Sounds sexist I know!).

SEX
Love and Health

As long as we are on the subject of things that feel good and are good for you, sex is an obvious gift from the gods. It's pretty simple to me—as long as it's consensual, it's a good thing. Sex and intimacy are incredible things and, ideally, you have both in your life. You don't need one to have the other; however, if you have both you are very fortunate.

From a purely primitive, physical perspective, I subscribe to the theory that, as in all body parts/functions, you either use it or lose it. Keep things flowing—just like the high volume dietary strategy.

Joseph J. Pizzorno, MD, CEO and Medical Director of Amai Wellness, says a good sex life is good for your heart. Sex also keeps your estrogen and testosterone levels in balance, helping to prevent problems like osteoporosis and heart disease. During one study, men who had sex at least twice a week were half as likely to die of heart disease as men who had sex rarely.

According to Mehmet Oz MD, Dr. Oz, professor of surgery and vice chairman of cardiovascular services at New York-Presbyterian/Columbia University, and co-author of *You on a Diet*, loving touches release hormones, including oxytocin, that reduce stress and anxiety. But if sex is a purely hedonistic process, it won't have the same results.

Keep Things Flowing
To ensure you keep things flowing, here are a few things you might want to explore:

Kegel Exercises for Men
The power of Kegel Exercises was shown in a 2005 British Study, BJU Int. 2005 Sep;96(4):595-7. After six months, 76% of men who made lifestyle changes such as stopping smoking, exercising, and losing weight had significantly improved their erectile dysfunction by including Kegel Exercises in their exercise routine. The improvement was much greater than the control group who had improved their lifestyle but not practiced Kegel Exercises. (https://www.ncbi.nlm.nih.gov/pmc/articles/PMC1324914/)

Pelvic floor muscle exercises for men:
In standing position:

Hardcore Health: Live Young!

Stand with your feet apart and tighten your pelvic floor muscles as if you were trying to stop the flow of urine and wind escaping. (Don't actually use the Kegel exercises to stop your urine flow as this can cause an infection.) If you look in a mirror, you should be able to see the base of your penis move nearer to your abdomen and your testicles rise.

Hold the contraction as strongly as you can.

Try to avoid holding your breath, pulling in your abdomen or tensing your buttocks.

Perform 3 maximal contractions in standing position, in the morning, holding 3 seconds.

Perform 3 maximal contractions in standing position, in the evening, holding for 3 seconds.

In sitting position:

Sit on a chair with your knees apart and tighten your pelvic floor muscles as if you were lifting your pelvic floor but not your buttocks off the chair.

Hold the contraction as strongly as you can.

Try to avoid holding your breath, pulling in your abdomen or tensing your buttocks.

Perform 3 maximal contractions while in sitting position, in the morning, holding for 3 seconds.

Perform 3 maximal contractions while in sitting position, in the evening, holding for 3 seconds.

In lying position:

Lie on your back with your knees bent and apart. Tighten your pelvic floor and hold the contraction as strongly as you can.

Try to avoid pulling in your abdomen or tensing your buttocks.

Perform 3 maximal contractions while in lying position, in the morning, holding for 3 seconds.

Perform 3 maximal contractions while in lying position, in the evening, holding for 3 seconds.

While walking, try lifting your pelvic floor up 50% of maximum.

After urinating, try tightening your pelvic floor muscles strongly to avoid the after-dribble.

During sexual activity, try tightening your pelvic floor muscles rhythmically to achieve and maintain penile rigidity. Slow thrusting movements generate higher pressures inside the penis.

To delay ejaculation:

For men with premature ejaculation, try tightening your pelvic floor muscles to delay ejaculation. In 1996, a study by the European Hospital in Rome, Italy found that Kegel Exercises help delay premature ejaculation.

Kegel Exercises may even boost libido.

And Memorial Sloan Kettering Cancer Center recommends Kegel Exercises for strengthening pelvic floor muscles and helping prevent urinary incontinence. In 2012, researchers found that a postoperative program including Kegel exercises improved men's ability to recover bladder control after prostate surgery. (https://www.mskcc.org/cancer-care/patient-education/pelvic-floor-muscle-kegel-exercises-women)

In order to find your pelvic muscles, The Center's advice is to imagine you are urinating and to contract the muscles you would need to stop the stream of urine. You can also tighten the muscles that you would use to hold back gas.

To do the Kegel Exercises, first empty your bladder. Then tighten your pelvic floor muscles for 2 to 3 seconds. Then relax the muscles completely for 10 seconds. Repeat this ten times. Repeat 7 to 10 times every day.

Kegel Exercises for Women

Research has found that toning the pelvic floor muscles can benefit sexual health and arousal. Kegel exercises can increase pelvic floor muscle strength and draw blood flow to the pelvic floor, which is important for arousal. Kegel exercises also help with bladder control and manage or prevent physical problems such as the leakage of urine.

To find your pelvic floor muscles, imagine you are urinating and contract the muscles you would need to stop the stream of urine. Do not actually practice stopping the urine stream as this could lead to a urinary tract infection. Then tighten the muscles that are used to hold back or prevent you from passing gas, but don't tighten your buttock or inner thigh muscles. If you're doing it correctly, there should be no visible movement of your body lifting. If you are tightening the muscles of your buttocks or abdomen, or notice that your body lifts slightly, you are most likely using the wrong muscles.

When doing Kegel Exercises, squeeze slowly and gently. Focus on feeling a squeeze which builds to a lifting sensation. Practice squeezing for a count of 5, then relaxing for a count of 5, repeat 10 times. Practice daily and as often as you like.

As a workout for improving sexual health and increasing libido, sexual health researchers recommend exercising your pelvic floor muscles with a series of exercises. First flex your urethra, the opening closest to the pubic bone. Then flex your vagina. Then move back and flex your anus. They recommend holding each flex for 3 to 5 seconds and repeating the sequence three times. Do three sets of three every day for a week. (https://newsinhealth.nih.gov/2018/03/power-pelvis) (https://www.niddk.nih.gov/health-information/urologic-diseases/bladder-control-problems-women/kegel-exercises)

Nitric Oxide and Sex

Hardcore Health: Live Young!

Nitric Oxide, a short-lived gas, is so beneficial to health that the Nobel Prize for Medicine was given to the group of scientists who discovered its medicinal properties and cardiovascular benefits. Nitric Oxide (NO) benefits the body by opening up blood vessels, increasing blood flow, giving you a better working heart and decreasing the chance of blood clotting. It is the neurotransmitter in the nerve cells that control erections.

Nitric oxide also helps transmit and process information between the nerve cells and the brain, therefore helping your memory become sharper. It assists the immune system in fighting off viruses and bacteria, improves immunity, regulates blood pressure, reduces inflammation on any part of the body, improves your quality of sleep, increases your sense of smell, and helps with endurance and strength. (You can read why Nitric Oxide researchers won the Nobel prize here: https://maximumcardio4u.com/nitric-oxid/)

Natural Sources of Nitric Oxide:
Natural sources are beet juice and foods containing the amino acids L-arginine and L-citrulline like nuts, green vegetables like spinach and arugula, some fruits like watermelon, and fish.

Exercise causes high levels of blood to pass through arterial walls and triggers nitric oxide to be released into the body. The harder you exercise, the better your cardiovascular health will get. When you run or lift weights, your muscles need more oxygen, which is supplied by the blood. Your heart will be able to pump blood more efficiently through your body and supply more oxygen to every part of your body much more efficiently by increasing nitrate oxide.

Ways to Stimulate Nitric Oxide
	Deep nasal breathing stimulates Nitric Oxide.
	Mehmet C. Oz M.D. (Dr. Oz) in his comprehensive book *You: Staying Young* says people with atherosclerosis (clogged and hardened arteries) commonly don't make enough nitric oxide to keep their arteries open. Nitrate oxide can influence whether you have a heart attack or suffer from erectile dysfunction. You can get it by meditation and breathing through your nose. Marathon runners breathe through their noses to keep blood moving through their bodies and stimulate nitric oxide. If you're overweight, you tend to breathe through your mouth when asleep and don't suck nitric oxide into your lungs, which can lead to sleep apnea and feeling tired and stressed. Lack of nitrate oxide can also lead to diabetes.
	Viagra and other impotence medications work due to their action on the nitric oxide pathway.

Viagra and Other Male Sexual Performance Drugs

Real Science Magazine, February 4, 2013, reports that, not only is Viagra extending men's sex lives, but clinical trials are underway using the little blue pill to fight obesity and cancer, including stopping the growth of pancreatic, stomach and prostate tumors, treat heart disease, widen arteries enough to lower blood pressure, improve circulation in fingers and toes, treat jet lag, diabetes symptoms, multiple sclerosis, chronic pelvic pain, and memory loss. (For details of this research see studies on Viagra in the August 2007 issue of Harvard Men's Health Watch. https://www.health.harvard.edu/newsletters/harvard_mens_health_watch/2007/august)

Viagra and other impotence medications work due to their action on the nitric oxide pathway. (See Nitric Oxide)

Sexy Foods

Some of my fondest and most fun sexual memories involve food products. See movie *9 1/2 Weeks* as an example, however in this case we are referring to digesting the food internally as opposed to simply using it as a topping (chocolate pudding and whip cream will never be the same)!

Fish: Wild Salmon, Albacore Tuna, Herring

Fatty fish that contain Omega-3 Fatty Acids help to raise dopamine levels.

Omega-3 fatty acids DHA and EPA found in fish help to raise dopamine levels in the brain that trigger arousal, according to sexologist Yvonne K. Fulbright, PhD. Other health benefits are the anti-inflammatory properties found in fish that fight blood clots and heart arrhythmias, improve brain function, and protection against dementia. Studies show that omega-3s can also reduce symptoms of depression. Research from the University of Pittsburgh shows that people with high omega-3 blood levels were happier and more agreeable.

Fish is also one of the many healthy foods that contain the amino acid L-arginine, which stimulates the release of growth hormone, among other substances, and is converted into nitric oxide in the body. Nitric oxide is critical for erections and it can help women's sexual function too by causing blood vessels to open wider for improved blood flow.

"Good fats" in fatty fish, like salmon and anchovies, also increase DHEA, a vital hormone made in the adrenal glands that usually peaks around the age of 25 and then declines over years.

A French study led by world-renowned neurosteroid researcher Étienne-Émile Baulieu reports that increasing levels of DHEA have a dramatic effect on libido, bone density and skin thickness for women over 69 years old. (See an interesting article at this link: http://www.life-enhancement.com/magazine/article/384-dhea-can-help-keep-women-in-love)

    Until DHEA supplementation is studied further, it would be safer to stick to natural sources of this hormone, as several studies have shown a positive correlation between DHEA supplementation and cancers of the prostate, ovaries and breast. Foods do not contain DHEA, but some foods might cause your body to produce more. DHEA is made from cholesterol, and your body makes cholesterol from healthy fats. You can get essential fatty acids from a variety of oils like ghee, raw butter, cod liver oil, coconut oil, red palm oil, flax seed oil, evening primrose oil, pumpkin seed and olive oils.

    One of the most effective ways to immediately boost your DHEA levels is to be touched, as in having a massage.

    Also, ensure you get plenty of sleep, preferably 7 – 8 hours a night.

    An anti-inflammatory diet is a critical part to de-stressing the body and boosting DHEA levels. This diet should be very low in sugar and carbohydrates and very rich in phytonutrients and trace minerals from fresh, raw or lightly steamed vegetables. Powerful anti-inflammatory herbs such as turmeric, ginger, rosemary, thyme, oregano, and cinnamon should be generously consumed on a regular basis to help the adrenal glands work more efficiently to produce more DHEA.

Watermelon

The production of dopamine also relies on vitamins and minerals, so make sure you eat plenty of fresh fruit and vegetables. Watermelon, which contains vitamins A, B6 and C, is a particularly good addition to the diet. Watermelon also contains beta-carotene, citrulline and lycopene, important phytonutrients for the heart and for sexual function.

According to studies at Texas A&M University, citrulline is particularly exciting for its ability to relax blood vessels. When you eat watermelon, the citrulline is converted to the helpful amino acid arginine. Arginine boosts nitric oxide, which relaxes blood vessels, the same basic effect that Viagra has, to treat erectile dysfunction and maybe even prevent it, according to Bhimu Patil PhD. Science Daily July, 2008 report (https://www.sciencedaily.com/releases/2008/06/080630165707.htm).

Red Wine

In a study reported in the *Journal of Sexual Medicine,* Oct 6, 2009, Italian researchers found that the antioxidants and polyphenols in red wine may trigger the production of nitric oxide in the blood, which helps artery walls to relax and widen, increasing blood flow to strategic places where you

Hardcore Health: Live Young!

probably want it to go. Nicola Mondaini, MD, advises sticking to one glass, as any more may extinguish your libido. Drinking a small amount of alcohol can also boost dopamine, which is why a glass of wine can help to put you in the mood.

Low-Fat Grass-Fed Beef, Lamb, Oysters
  Low-fat grass-fed beef is a great source of zinc, the same libido-boosting nutrient found in oysters. Zinc increases your testosterone and curbs production of prolactin, a hormone that can impair sexual function. Oysters are an aphrodisiac because they are high in zinc. Other foods high in zinc include meat, eggs, seafood and tofu.
  A study in the *Journal of the American College of Nutrition*, Oct 4, 2000, of varsity football players at Western Washington University found that supplements of 30 mg. zinc, 450 mg magnesium, and Vitamin B-6 increased levels of testosterone.
(https://www.ncbi.nlm.nih.gov/pubmed/1619184)

Wheat Germ and L-arginine
  Wheat Germ, for those who aren't gluten sensitive, is rich in L-arginine, which can be found in energy supplements. Wheat germ is the small, reproductive part of the wheat kernel that germinates and develops into wheat grass. This kernel, which includes the wheat germ, is unfortunately removed during the refining of whole

wheat grains to white flour because its healthy oils become rancid quickly. The germ itself only makes up about 3% of the kernel, and you need over 50 pounds of wheat to get one pound of wheat germ.

According to Leslie Bonci, M.P.H., R.D., CSSD, Director Sports Nutrition Program at the University of Pittsburgh Medical Center, L-arginine is a vasodilator, sometimes called 'Athlete's Viagra'. It increases oxygen delivery to all organs of the body. (For more sports nutrition advice see website: https://activeeatingadvice.com/)

Wheat germ is also an excellent source of zinc, a mineral that is often associated with sexual health and improved erectile function. Zinc is found in high concentrations in the prostate, which indicates it is critical for proper function of the prostate gland. Zinc also helps increase blood flow. Wheat germ contains more nutrients (23) per ounce than any other grain or vegetable. In addition to zinc, wheat germ is high in protein, potassium and magnesium (both important for blood pressure and the heart), iron, riboflavin, calcium, and vitamins A, B1, B3, and E. Athletes use wheat germ to improve cardiovascular function.

Wheat germ can be sprinkled on cereals, casseroles, smoothies, baked goods, grains, salads, and vegetables.

Flaxseed, Granola, Cashews—Other Sources of L-argentine

If you need to avoid gluten-containing ingredients but would like to benefit from the flavor and nutritional value of wheat germ, you have a few substitutes that may work. Ground flaxseed meal is nutty and can provide a satisfying texture and color to baked foods. Ground almond meal serves as a good source for vitamin E and protein, two nutrients provided by wheat germ. The Gluten Intolerance Group considers both safe. L-arginine is also found in granola, cashews, pistachios, watermelon and root vegetables.

Those who are gluten intolerant should check ingredient labels to ensure that foods aren't made in facilities where gluten-containing foods are also processed, since this could contaminate the food with gluten.

Spinach

According to *The Women's Health Big Book of Sex,* spinach is a potent source of magnesium, which helps dilate blood vessels, according to Japanese researchers. Better blood flow to the genitals creates greater arousal for men and women.

Protein—Meat, Fish, Chicken, Eggs

Animal fat encourages the production of sex hormones and having a good balance of hormones is essential to a healthy sex life. According to Dr Cecilia Tregear, President of the British Society of Anti-Aging Medicine, it's vital to eat plenty of good quality protein, ideally a portion with every meal. A good balance of animal fat in meat, chicken and fish and good cholesterol found in eggs, for example, encourages the production of sex hormones, improving libido,

BENEFITS OF PHYSICAL LABOR

Another way to maintain your body is through menial tasks and physical labor, including fine motor skills. You should never think you are above putting in a hard day's physical work, whether it be cleaning your yard or scrubbing your floors. There is something zen about hard physical labor using repetitive motions. It may not sound sexy, but it is very fulfilling—especially when you have finished a massive task and can cool down and admire your work, whether it's a manicured lawn or shiny house. This kind of work also keeps you honest and makes you appreciate the fact that you don't have to put in hard labor to make a living (unless of course you do and in that case, I recommend the opposite type of work to mix it up).

It's also useful if you can fix or construct things that are small and require using your fine motor skills. It is important to use all parts of your body and use them in all ways possible. After all, your fingers were designed to not only hold onto large things but also to perform pinpoint operations that require concentration and careful micro maneuvers. I find it very rewarding when, after

Hardcore Health: Live Young!

spending a day completing a fine motor skill task, my hands and fingers actually hurt a little the next day. I interpret that as having exercised and utilized some of the equipment that has been getting a free ride.

REHAB

There is a classic line in the movie *One Flew Over the Cuckoo's Nest* where Jack Nicholson's character takes the mentally challenged Martini (Danny DeVito) out on a fishing boat and puts a rod in his hand and says, "You're a fisherman, Martini!"

We are what we think we are. I think of myself as an aging world-class athlete. I surf big North Shore waves at 50+, so that puts me in a very small subset of people. Therefore, if I consider myself a world-class athlete, I should train and eat like one. Along those same lines, if I get injured I have to rehabilitate myself as quickly and efficiently as possible to get myself back into the game.

I believe in a very simple principle—we have four limbs (two arms/two legs) and if one is injured, work the other three harder or at least the opposite two. For instance, if I have a mild shoulder separation, I work my lower body (legs) harder. If you see me out of the water and not paddling for a few days, but rather riding up the volcano on my bike, you could guess that I hurt my shoulder. On the other hand, if you see me only paddling and not running errands on my bike, you can bet I hurt my knee. Note that I usually take a few rounds of Advil/Ibuprofen during these rehab periods.

Either way, the strategy is to rest the injured body part, if it is more than just a slight sprain, for a day or two and focus on the other limbs. After a few days, I ease back into strengthening the injured body part by light paddling or biking.

Again the focus is on being ready for the game or the next big swell, so I'll typically rest and rehab as determined from the surf forecast. If I know I have a week before the next big swell, I can take my time. Of course if the injury is really bad, I will rest it completely and that sometimes includes shutting all the limbs down for a few days. This also makes for a good recharge of the body. I also try to sleep and stay horizontal as much as possible during these rehab stints. Your body will usually indicate to you what it needs.

My overall philosophy, however, is to always work through mild to moderate injuries. Again, use it or lose it and keep it moving. If you take months off from physical activity, it is going to be really hard to get back into it, especially if you are a senior citizen!

SLEEP AS FUEL

Sleep is critical for your body to recharge after your daily physical and mental activities. A lot of people have trouble going to sleep because they bombard their senses with electronic stimuli like TV, video, and the internet prior to going to bed. It seems to make more sense to wind down by reading a book, listening to some relaxing music, taking a walk outside (dogs are useful for this purpose as they need to go out) to reset your mind to what ideally will be the peaceful experience of sleep.

    I was not a good sleeper as a kid. My mind was always racing on what I had to do the next day in school or reviewing what transpired that day. What helped me through those long nights was Sports Talk Radio. Larry King started his career as a sports radio host and his monotone voice helped me get through many a sleep-challenged night when I was a little kid. Even though we are way into the 21st century, I still enjoy radio as a medium. It's a little like reading a book. You picture what is happening in your mind and sharpen your creativity as opposed to seeing the pictures on TV or video, where you are subjected to someone else's vision of the words. This is why books are almost always better than the movie versions of a good story.

    In regard to using the sports talk radio as a sleep incentive, there are two ways to approach the problem:

        1. Listen to the content and let your mind wander on these mild sports topics; or
        2. Keep the radio on a volume that is barely discernible to create a pleasant background

noise like a humming ceiling fan so your mind doesn't focus on the issues being discussed. This could also work with audio books. In a related example, babies spend 9 months in their mom's belly's listening to the swooshing sound of amniotic fluid around them and that is why they design crib audio baby devices that mimic that sound. (It worked well with my kids.)

Another trick, conveyed to me by no doubt desperate parents when I was a kid trying to get to sleep, was that if you are lying down with your eyes closed, it is almost as good as sleeping. I think this was just a distraction technique they used to get me to mellow out, but the result was often positive in that I would at least lay there for an hour or two with my eyes closed, relaxing and in position to fall asleep eventually.

The bottom line is: get as much sleep as you can, even if you have to fake it and just relax and tell yourself you are sleeping. I shoot for 6- 8 hours a night if I am lucky and I know how much better my body and mind feel after a good night's sleep.

Dr. Florence Comite, of the Comite Center for Precision Medicine, a leader in the field of personalized medicine, says that adequate sleep is by far and away the number one thing that trumps everything else when it comes to healthy aging. Although we live in a society where it's common to burn the candles at both ends and think it's perfectly fine to have five or six hours of sleep and that's enough, sleep is critical for health. Sleep deprivation is associated with diabetes, heart disease, obesity, high blood pressure, and other conditions. During sleep, the immune system activates and the body heals from the damages of the day.

During deep sleep—what we call slow-wave sleep—human growth hormone is released, according to sleep expert Phil Gehrman PhD. Sleep is part of normal tissue repair, patching the wear and tear of the day. This hormone promotes growth when we are young. As we age, it helps increase muscle mass, thicken skin and strengthen bones.

Research shows that people who sleep fewer than five or six hours a night tend to age faster. Chronic sleep loss can lead to lackluster skin, fine lines, and dark circles under the eyes. With lack of sleep, more of the stress hormone cortisol is released and this can break down skin collagen.

Sleep Sabotages
The following foods are best avoided near bedtime:
Caffeine: Coffee, some sodas, dark chocolate (not white chocolate), hot cocoa and tea, as all contain caffeine that can keep you awake.
Fatty foods: Foods high in fat and fried foods take longer to digest and interfere with sleep.
Heavy meals: Steak, roast beef, and protein-rich foods are slow to digest and disturb sleep

Foods rich in Tyramine: Tomatoes, eggplant, soy sauce, red wine, aged cheeses such as Brie and Stilton contain tyramine, an amino acid that triggers the brain to release norepinephrine, a stimulant that interferes with sleep.

Bean dishes, chili: The body has a hard time digesting beans and causes gas that disturbs sleep. (My body has acclimatized itself to beans. Fortunately!)

Broccoli: Broccoli, cauliflower and brussel sprouts are slow to digest and can cause gas that can keep you awake at night.

Sleep Enhancers
Omega-3

Michael Breuss PhD, the Sleep doctor, says that 99% of women lack omega-3s and sleep issues are a sign of a shortage. The body needs omega-3s to produce melatonin. He recommends eating one serving of foods rich in omega 3 fatty acids daily (salmon, flaxseeds, eggs) and supplementing with 185 mg of EPA and 115 mg of DHA found in fish oil capsules.

Blood Glucose

Low blood glucose triggers nighttime awakenings. Ronald Hoffman, M.D. of the Hoffman Center, New York recommends eating a snack like an apple with peanut butter 30 minutes before bed.

Magnesium

A Dec 20, 2012 study in the *Journal of Research in Medical Sciences* found that people who supplemented with magnesium saw a threefold improvement in sleep efficiency (time spent sleeping rather than lying awake). Replenishing magnesium can calm the adrenal glands and stop them pumping out stress hormone cortisol.

SLEEP AID

Ingredients:
1 tbsp coconut oil
1/4 tsp raw honey
1/8 tsp sea salt or pink Himalayan salt

Combine your coconut oil and honey in a small bowl, then stir in some salt. Stir until well combined. Take a spoonful with some water.

The combination of these ingredients sets your body in its 'sleeping mode.' It normalizes the secretion of stress hormones and keeps your cortisol spikes under control. It is actually the spikes that wake you up at 3am. Coconut oil prevents a blood glucose spike, which are another major cause of insomnia.

Honey does not affect your blood sugar and it provides the proper amount of the glycogen that your brain needs. Insufficient glycogen levels stimulate your adrenals to produce more stress hormones. High levels of stress hormones keep you awake at night.

Salt decreases the secretion of adrenaline and cortisol.

PERPETUAL WORKING

The old model used to be work hard and retire when you are around 60 years old, however that seems to be backwards to me as I have seen many people retire and then become depressed and even die! If possible, if you can make your work your passion, then you never need or want to retire. Of course you may need or want to slow down; however, working into extreme old age is a good thing if you can pull it off. Just as in *Hardcore Inventing,* we advise not quitting your day job until you can quit and achieve self-employed financially independent inventor status. If you can achieve that status with your passion as your work, then let that become your lifelong perpetual working model.

Perpetual working into old age is not just good for the obvious reasons of providing cash flow to support you as you strive for 100 years of age, it can keep you sharp mentally and help avoid Alzheimer's and other ailments of the mind. (Use it or lose it applies here too!)

Ideally, your perpetual-motion, self-employed, passion/career will include mental challenges, physical challenges, and fine-motor skills components. If you can create a home business and keep your overhead razor thin, then you can optimize your potential to be profitable.

Hardcore Health: Live Young!

And even if you only break even monetarily, you are still greatly benefiting from the mental and physical exercise and engagement.

You may be monetarily set from your real/early life's work, however it might be good to get involved in a "cause" where you become a home-based activist or volunteer. Although money is not the objective of this activity, you can check the other boxes relative to keeping your mind and body engaged.

A University of Maryland study discovered that people who work part-time after they retire have fewer chronic diseases and physical limitations. And recent French research shows that people who retire earlier have an increased risk for Alzheimer's disease.

There needs to be a sense of fulfillment, if possible. That is why it is important to figure out what makes you happy in your work and your resulting accomplishments. It may be building a device with your own hands that you sell to your customers or it could be helping people with their problems. This is a very personal choice that you have to figure out yourself. Later in life there may be a chance to engage in a career, at least on a volunteer basis, that you always wanted to try out but never could, given life's circumstances. Working or volunteering also help keep you active and not a couch potato; though, unfortunately, many office jobs also involve too much sitting.

In a 2015 issue of the *British Journal of Sports Medicine*, British experts warn about the dangers of prolonged sitting. They recommend office workers stand for at least two hours a day, adding they should eventually double that to four hours.

Add action to your working day by stretching, standing during phone calls, holding walking meetings. Take walks during lunch time, use the stairs instead of the elevators.

CHAPTER 2—FIGHT DISEASE WITH DIET AND LIFESTYLE

FIGHT CANCER WITH DIET AND LIFESTYLE

Being diagnosed with cancer has to be one of the worst health issues we can encounter. My mother had that misfortune and it was a bad one—Stage 4 Non-Hodgkin's Lymphoma. We were all devastated, but not my mom. She fought it head on with her team of doctors and with my father coaching her through it.

One of the key decisions she made was not to stay put in her hometown with her local oncologist, but instead to search out the cancer institute in the country that had seen the most cases of her type of cancer. This is a key strategy that I have seen work repeatedly. It doesn't make sense to stay with only your local oncologist who has seen only a handful of Stage 4 Non-Hodgkin's Lymphoma vs. a cancer research institute that has seen thousands of that particular type of cancer.

Not only was the center they chose extremely well-versed in that type of cancer, but they were a research institute so they were always on the cutting edge of trying new approaches. MD Anderson in Houston was the institute that my mom chose to start her battle. Note that she did not insult or disregard her local oncologist, but rather kept them on as her local Florida team.

At MD Anderson in Houston, the experienced staff immediately recognized the dire state that my mother was in relative to the progression of her cancer and started her on an aggressive course of chemotherapy. It saved her life! They also tried some experimental interferon (a biological) to combat the cancer as they were not simply going to rely on chemotherapy alone.

My mom, with the encouragement of my father, also undertook a multi-pronged approach to her healing, including fine-tuning her diet with healthier food with more veggies and fiber and meditation/positive-thinking. She lost her hair as was expected, but kept fighting all along. It seems to me that the battle to survive in the case of cancer fighters is similar to lost-at-sea survivors (e.g., Louie Zamperini of *Unbroken* fame) —the mind battle is an important component to assure victory, the fight is not just on the physical front. My mom was all-in on fighting the cancer chemically, physically, mentally— whatever it took to beat it down!

Twenty-seven years later, my mom is a proud cancer survivor! She fought hard and it didn't get the best of her. She still goes back to MD Anderson a few times a year to check on the status and ensure the cancer is not trying to make a comeback.

The key to her survival was venturing out to get multiple opinions and tracking down the experts in the country (or world if necessary) to help treat the cancer she was dealing with, combined with her determination to survive and fight.

    Chemotherapy is still a mainstay of cancer treatment, but the hottest frontier is immunotherapy—tapping into the body's immune system to attack tumors. Immunotherapy drugs are credited with helping treat former President Jimmy Carter's advanced melanoma. The approach was pioneered by MD Anderson immunologist, Jim Allison. (Read more at: https://www.mdanderson.org/cancermoonshots/research_platforms/immunotherapy.html) The drugs have worked well with some melanoma and lung cancer and are now being explored for a wide variety of tumors. (https://www.ncbi.nlm.nih.gov/pubmed/29254498)

    Analysts predict that in 10 years, Immunotherapy will be used to treat as many as 60 percent of people with advanced cancer. To that end, about 500 trials are underway around the nation testing checkpoint inhibitors against 32 cancers, most finding benefit in some patients. More than 100 of the trials are being conducted at MD Anderson, 32 in the lung, head and neck department alone. Research includes "basket trials," which group different cancers, testing the premise that checkpoint inhibitors treat a patient's immune system, not the cancer. One checkpoint inhibitor, given for any cancer that had spread or was otherwise considered incurable, including kidney, colon and a number of stomach tumors, produced positive responses in a fifth of 140 patients.

A unique, noninvasive, multi-analyte blood test that screens for eight common cancer types has been developed by Johns Hopkins Kimmel Cancer Center researchers. The test called CancerSEEK evaluates levels of eight cancer proteins and the presence of cancer gene mutations from circulating DNA. It also helps identify the location of the cancer. The findings were published online by *Science* on Jan. 18, 2018. Ovary, liver, esophagus, pancreas, stomach, colorectal, lung, and breast cancer. (Read more at: https://www.nih.gov/news-events/nih-research-matters/blood-test-detects-several-cancer-types)

A larger-scale trial must be done before CancerSEEK can be made commercially available, and a new study featuring 10,000 healthy individuals is underway.

Fight Prostate Cancer

Other than skin cancer, prostate cancer is the most common cancer in American men. The American Cancer Society's estimates for prostate cancer in the United States for 2015 are about 220,800 new cases of prostate cancer and about 27,540 deaths from prostate cancer. Can diet help or prevent prostate cancer?

Hardcore Health: Live Young!

A 2009 review published in the *Journal of Human Nutrition and Dietetics* assessed whether certain modifications in diet have a beneficial effect on the prevention of prostate cancer. Results suggest that a diet low in fat, red meat, dairy, and calcium yet high in fruits and green vegetables and tomatoes is beneficial in preventing and treating prostate cancer. Consumption of highly processed or charcoaled meats, dairy products and fats seemed to be correlated with prostate cancer. (https://www.ncbi.nlm.nih.gov/pubmed/19344379)

Research findings published in the Jan 11, 2005 *Journal of Nutritional Biochemistry* indicate that nutrients in avocados inhibit the growth of prostate cancer cells. Researchers at UCLA discovered that avocados are the richest source of lutein among commonly eaten fruits. Lutein is a carotenoid that acts as an antioxidant. It has been linked to a reduced risk of prostate cancer in previous studies. A Jun 12, 2013 *Harvard-based Health Professionals Follow-up Study* suggests that limiting animal fats and eating more healthy vegetable fats like avocado, walnuts, extra virgin olive oil can help fight the disease. (Read the study on avocado at :https://www.ncbi.nlm.nih.gov/pmc/articles/PMC3664913/)

Evidence suggests taking a low-dose aspirin (81 milligrams) daily may protect you from developing many types of cancer, including those hardest to treat successfully, says Robert S. Bresalier, M.D. Hepatology and Nutrition at MD Anderson. Prostrate cancer, breast cancer, colon cancer and rectal cancer are among the most common and life-threatening cancers in the United States, according to the National Cancer Institute. Aspirin use could have a positive impact on your risks for these diseases. Aspirin reduces the risk of cancer by fighting inflammation, Dr. Bresalier says. Aspirin blocks the production of the enzymes that increase inflammation in your body and speed or assist the growth of cancer cells. Ultimately, this helps lower your cancer risks or slows the spread of the disease. (https://www.mdanderson.org/publications/focused-on-health/november-2014/low-dose-aspirin-cancer-prevention.html)

    A daily low-dose aspirin may make sense for people at high risk for certain types of cancer, but the drug's potential side effects mean aspirin certainly isn't for everyone.

    In his book *Earl Mindell's Supplement Bible*, Earl Mindell R.Ph, PhD. suggests part of the reason American men are five times more likely than Japanese men to die from prostate cancer could be diet. The Asian diet contains four times the amount of selenium as the average American diet.

    Much of the food sold in grocery sores is highly processed, making it difficult for Americans to get enough selenium. Dr. Andrew Weil in Ask Dr.

Weil says eating just one shelled Brazil nut—grown in the selenium-rich soil of central Brazil—provides 120 micrograms of the mineral, getting you that much closer to the daily target of 200 micrograms.

India has one of the lowest rates of prostate cancer in the world. Most Indian food contains the yellow spice turmeric with the active ingredient curcumin, which is a powerful antioxidant for men. Studies show the spice may help fight prostate cancer as well as Alzheimer's disease, arthritis, and Parkinson's disease. (https://www.ncbi.nlm.nih.gov/pmc/articles/PMC4060744/)

The new study from a German Research team headed by Dr. Beatrice Bachmeier at Ludwig-Maximilians-Universitat in Munich found that curcumin reduces the expression of two pro-inflammatory proteins involved in prostate cancer, and in mice curcumin caused a reduction in the incidences of metastases. Bachmeier has suggested curcumin may help prevent prostate cancers and stop their ability to spread. She warned it should not be seen as a replacement for conventional therapies.

A Feb 10, 2012 study from Thomas Jefferson University found that curcumin might help slow the progression of tumor growth in men with hormone-resistant prostate cancer. Curcumin increased the results of hormone therapy, reduced the number of prostate cancer cells when compared with hormone therapy alone and inhibited the cell cycle and survival of prostate cancer cells.

Fight Colon Cancer

Colorectal cancer is the third most common type of cancer diagnosed in the U.S., excluding skin cancers, according to the American Cancer Society.

Dr. Michael Orlich, of Loma Linda University in California, and colleagues looked at 77,695 Seventh-Day Adventist men and women who have been taking part in a long-term study of health and diet. Seventh-Day Adventists are encouraged to eat a healthy diet and avoid smoking and other unhealthy habits. Many are vegetarian or vegan, but some eat fish and some eat certain meats such as chicken or lamb.

Over seven years, vegans and vegetarians had about a 22 percent lower risk of colorectal cancer, Orlich's team reported in the *Journal of the American Medical Association's* JAMA's Internal Medicine. Reduction in meat intake may be a primary reason for the reduced risk demonstrated in vegetarians, but an increase in the consumption of various whole plant foods might also contribute to the reduction.
(https://www.ncbi.nlm.nih.gov/pmc/articles/PMC4420687/)

The National Heart, Lung and Blood Institute state that a low-fat plant based diet would not only lower the heart attack rate by about 85%

but would also lower the cancer rate by 60%. People who ate fish but not meat seemed to have the lowest risk of colon cancer—43% lower than people who ate meat. Orlich's team says the omega-3 fatty acids in fish may be responsible. Vegetarian sources include walnuts and flaxseed oil.

Cancer fighters that scientists recommend adding to your diet include olive oil; tomato sauce—the type you find with pasta—containing the carotenoid lycopene; liver detoxers like broccoli, broccoli sprouts, and dark greens; green tea, which has high antioxidant polyphenols; and B vitamins including folate.

Frank Garland MD recommends Vitamin D in the prevention and fights against colon cancer. (https://www.ncbi.nlm.nih.gov/pmc/articles/PMC1470481/)

Evidence suggests taking a low-dose aspirin (81 milligrams) daily reduces the risk of colorectal cancer. Part of this reduction in risk might be due to protection against metastatic disease. (https://www.ncbi.nlm.nih.gov/pmc/articles/PMC5590216/)

Low doses of aspirin or "baby aspirin" are generally 81 milligrams in the United States (100 milligrams in Europe), while a regular-strength adult aspirin is typically 325 milligrams.

A daily low-dose aspirin may make sense for people at high risk for certain types of cancer, but the drug's potential side effects mean aspirin certainly isn't for everyone.

Researchers from Linus Pauling Institute conducted research in 2007 showing just how powerful the sulforaphane in cruciferous vegetables is. They found that, as powerful as broccoli is, broccoli sprouts are 50 times more packed with sulforaphane. Broccoli sprouts are also recommended to help with liver detox and improve liver health, which helps fight many forms of cancer including colon cancer. (http://lpi.oregonstate.edu/mic/food-beverages/cruciferous-vegetables)

Broccoli sprouts are also in a trial against advanced pancreatic cancer. (https://www.ncbi.nlm.nih.gov/pmc/articles/PMC4059031/)

Fight Lung Cancer

The American Cancer Society states that the best way to reduce your risk of lung cancer is not to smoke and to avoid breathing in other people's smoke. Some evidence suggests that a diet high in fruits and vegetables may help protect against lung cancer in both smokers and non-smokers, but any positive effect of fruits and vegetables on lung cancer risk would be much less than the increased risk from smoking. If you stop smoking before a cancer develops, your damaged lung tissue gradually starts to repair itself. No matter what your

Hardcore Health: Live Young!

age or how long you've smoked, quitting may lower your risk of lung cancer and help you live longer.

Tips to Quit Smoking

Addictions are hard to beat. But you can do it. Here are some tips from the experts:

Create a plan.

Set a date and throw away your cigarettes and ashtrays.

If smoking is part of your routine, change it. Instead of lighting up after a meal, go for a walk or do something else that you enjoy instead.

Seek support. Tell friends and family that you are quitting smoking and ask them to help you stay accountable. Maybe they will quit too and you can do it as a team.

Get expert help. Your doctor can recommend medications and patches. Or call a helpline like 800-QUIT-NOW.

Exercise. Physical activity eases the symptoms of nicotine withdrawal, helps relieve stress, limits weight gain and improves lung function. Try something you enjoy like walking, swimming, dancing or kickboxing.

Foods that May Help Inhibit Tumor Growth:

The compounds described have shown promising results against lung cancer in-vitro and in-vivo.

(https://www.ncbi.nlm.nih.gov/pmc/articles/PMC4409137/)

Green Tea, derived from the plant Camellia sinensis, is the most common beverage consumed globally. Significant data from various studies provide evidence that tea consumption has a preventive effect on carcinogenesis.

Indol-3-carbinol is an autolysis product of glucosinolate present in Brassica plants like cabbage, cauliflower, kale, broccoli, brussel sprouts and has been reported to have anticancer effects.

Genistein (4,5,7-trihydroxyisoflavone), the most abundant isoflavone in soybean, has been widely reported for its chemopreventive and chemotherapeutic effects.

Curcumin (diferuloylmethane), derived from the plant Curcuma longa, has been widely studied for its antioxidant, antiangiogenic, analgesic, anti-inflammatory, and antiseptic properties. Treatment with curcumin (0.6%) decreased the expression of COX-2 in subcutaneous tumors in-vivo and led to decrease in weight of intralung tumors accompanied by an increase in survival rate.

Pomegranate: In athymic nude mice implanted with human lung cancer A549 cells, oral administration of PFE caused significant inhibition of tumor growth, and the latency period for the appearance of small solid tumors was prolonged in animals.

Fisetin (3,3',4',7-tetrahydroxyflavone) is a naturally occurring flavonoid and is found in strawberry, persimmon, grape, apple, cucumber and onion. It has antiproliferative, apoptotic and antiagiogenic properties in cancer cells.

Fight Breast Cancer

Breast Cancer is the most common cancer among women in both developed and less-developed countries. The World Cancer Research Fund (WCRF) and American Cancer Society (ACS) cancer prevention guidelines recommend maintaining a healthy weight, limiting alcohol, avoiding smoking, staying physically active, limiting medical imaging with high exposure to radiation like tomography, and avoiding environmental pollution such as workplace pollution, gas fumes and vehicle exhaust fumes. (https://www.wcrf.org/int/research-we-fund/our-cancer-prevention-recommendations)

A low-fat diet appears to offer a slight reduction in the risk of breast cancer. A healthy diet may decrease your risk of other types of cancer, as well as diabetes, heart disease and stroke. Cancer fighting foods that scientists recommend adding to your diet include olive oil; tomato sauce—the type you find with pasta—containing the carotenoid lycopene; liver detoxers like broccoli, broccoli sprouts and dark greens, green tea, which has high antioxidant polyphenols; plus B vitamins including folate and Vitamin D.

Choose hormone-free dairy and animal products such as organic chicken, grass-fed beef and organic produce.

Dr. Joseph Pizzorno N.D., founding president of Bastyr University and author of *The Encyclopedia of Natural Medicine,* says that Breast Cancer risk is largely a result of diet and lifestyle.

Dietary factors include: body weight, increased intake of saturated fats, decreased intake of anti-oxidants, dietary fiber, omega 3 fatty acids (particularly alpha-linolenic acid), and dietary phytoestrogens (estrogen-like compounds found in foods such as legumes, nuts and seeds). Dr. Pizzorno recommends following the Mediterranean diet.

Environmental factors include: lack of exercise, alcohol consumption, smoking.

Andrew Weil, MD, www.drweil.com, warns that a large number of synthetic chemical compounds have estrogen-like activity. These include common pesticides, industrial pollutants and hormone residues in meat, poultry and dairy products. While evidence linking these hormones to breast cancer is conflicting, Dr. Weil recommends limiting exposure as much as possible

According to research by Drs. Frank and Cedric Garland and colleagues, UC San Diego School of Medicine and Moores Cancer Center, optimizing your vitamin D levels could help you to prevent several types of cancer including breast, colorectal, ovarian, and prostate. (https://health.ucsd.edu/news/releases/Pages/2016-04-06-low-vitamin-d-higher-cancer-risk.aspx.) Further studies recommend vitamin D be obtained through diet and exposure to sunlight. Foods with some vitamin D are fatty fish, fish liver oil, egg yolks, fortified milk and cereals.

    A study in the *Journal of Clinical Oncology*, Mar 20, 2010, of recovering breast cancer patients found that those who took a daily aspirin for three to five years were 60% less likely to suffer from a recurrence of the disease. The aspirin takers also were 71% less likely to die as a result of cancer. (https://www.ncbi.nlm.nih.gov/pubmed/20159825)

    Recently, a study in the *British Journal of Nutrition* showed that pairing broccoli with a spice containing the enzyme myrosinase seemed to enhance broccoli's cancer-fighting benefits. To get this effect, Elizabeth Jeffery PhD, Professor Emerita of Nutrition and Professor Emerita of Pharmacology at the University of Illinois, recommends spicing up your broccoli and broccoli sprouts with mustard, horseradish, or wasabi.

    Alcohol is linked to an increased risk of developing breast cancer. The risk increases with the amount of alcohol consumed. Compared with non-drinkers, women who consume one alcoholic drink a day have a very small increase in risk.

Those who have two to five drinks daily have about 1½ times the risk of women who don't drink alcohol. Excessive alcohol consumption is also known to increase the risk of developing several other types of cancer.

Stay Physically Active
Physical activity of at least three hours moderate aerobic-type activity a week—brisk walking, swimming or dancing—is recommended.

Physical activity after a breast cancer diagnosis may lower the risk of death from that disease. The benefit was seen particularly among women who had tumors over-expressing estrogen receptors and progesterone receptors. These results are consistent with a hormonal mechanism. The maximum benefit occurred among women who performed the equivalent of walking three to five hours per week at an average pace (2-2.9 mph). (See more benefits of physical activity: https://www.ncbi.nlm.nih.gov/pmc/articles/PMC3490043/#S5title)

Watch Your Weight
Overweight and obese women have a higher risk of being diagnosed with breast cancer compared to women who maintain a healthy weight, especially after menopause. Being overweight also can increase the risk of the breast cancer recurring in women who have had the disease. This higher

risk is because fat cells make estrogen, extra fat cells mean more estrogen in the body, and estrogen can make hormone-receptor-positive breast cancers develop and grow.

To Lose Weight:

Limit sugar and refined carbohydrates like white bread, cake, and alcohol.

Eat small portions. Fill two-thirds of your plate with fresh organic vegetables, fruits, and whole grains and one-third or less with meat and dairy products.

Choose non-fat milk and dairy products.

Drink water or drinks with no sugar. Avoid soda, lemonade, sweetened iced tea, and juices.

Keep healthy snacks on hand such as carrot and celery sticks (organic is best), non-fat Greek or plain yogurt, apple slices (organic is best), orange sections, air-popped (without butter) popcorn, unsweetened tea or herbal tea.

Fight Skin Cancer

To protect yourself from skin cancer, follow these tips:

Avoid the sun during the middle of the day.

Wear sunscreen, apply generously. Zinc or a SPF of at least 15.

Wear protective clothing with long sleeves and a broad-rimmed hat. Wear sunglasses.

Avoid tanning beds.

Beware of sun sensitizing medications. Ask your doctor if the medication you are taking makes you more sensitive to sunlight.

Check your skin regularly and report suspicious changes to your doctor.

The Dana-Farber/Brigham and Women's Cancer Center Blog Jun 29, 2015 reports that studies have found that higher intake of retinol-rich foods, such as fish, milk, eggs, dark green leafy vegetables, and orange/yellow fruits and vegetables led to a 20% reduced risk of developing melanoma. Studies also show selenium-rich diets, with foods such as Brazil nuts, scallops, and barley, may reduce risk and support surviving the disease. Green tea shows possible benefits. (http://blog.dana-farber.org/insight/2015/06/what-is-the-link-between-diet-and-melanoma/)

The National Center for Complementary and Integrative Health recommends getting antioxidants from foods instead of supplements as previous studies have linked high dose supplements to increased risk of certain cancers and diabetes. (https://nccih.nih.gov/health/antioxidants/introduction.htm)

Low blood levels of vitamin D have been associated with an increased risk for developing melanoma and worse survivorship outcomes. It's important to note that more is not always better; benefits do not continue to increase infinitely with more vitamin D intake, and there are risks associated with excessive vitamin D levels. Keep an open conversation with your doctor about any vitamins or supplements you plan to take. (https://www.ncbi.nlm.nih.gov/pmc/articles/PMC3897580/)

Sunscreen

Make sure you apply sunscreen every time you go outside, even if it is cloudy. When people tell me they don't need sunscreen because it's not sunny outside, my standard reply is that if there was no sun, it would be dark. In fact, some of the worst sunburns I've seen were acquired on cloudy days.

Make sure you cover your skin completely with sunscreen. I learned a great lesson in my teens from my friend's father who wore a long-sleeve white shirt in the middle of the day in blazing sun and heat. I finally figured out that the white long-sleeve shirts keep the sun off your entire arm (no truck driver's tan) and the color white has the highest reflectivity rate and therefore keeps you cool. It's like wearing an umbrella. Again looking to nature, the Bedouins roam the desert for years, but you don't see them wearing tank tops—they are always completely covered!

If, like me, you like your skin to completely take in the sun and water (in small doses, during my one hour paddle event), you have to figure out a way to cover the middle of your back with sunscreen. I was forced to solve this problem after a dermatologist dug a pre-cancerous lump out of the middle of my back and told me I have to cover and protect this area.

I don't have an adoring fan base around me at all times to apply sunscreen, and the one time I asked a friend to do it, I had, in turn, to apply it to his back. I can honestly say that I am not into applying sunscreen to a guy's hairy back, so I had to come up with an invention to solve this problem. I put on my primitive inventing cap and came up with a simple solution that, aside from being slightly embarrassing to an observer, is extremely effective. Go to a hardware store and buy a small paint roller pad with an extension handle and paint your middle back with sunscreen and you will avoid the sunburned middle back problem.

Marina Peredo, MD, Associate Clinical Professor of Dermatology at Mount Sinai Hospital, New York, warns that men are more likely than women to be diagnosed with skin cancer. Men do not apply sun protection as routinely as women and tend to spend more time outdoors. They may not visit a dermatologist regularly for a yearly skin cancer body check, which would help detect any abnormalities and precancerous lesions on the skin. Dermatologist Whitney Bowie, MD, says melanoma can occur anywhere on the body, but it's most likely to occur on the trunk in men.

Does Sunscreen Help you Look Younger?

Hardcore Health: Live Young!

Sunscreen protects against skin cancer, but does using it make you look younger? In a study published in the *Annals of Internal Medicine*, researchers at the Queensland Institute of Medical Research at the University of Queensland, Australia, examined 903 people 55 and younger to see whether daily sunscreen would stall aging. (http://annals.org/aim/article-abstract/1691733/sunscreen-prevention-skin-aging-randomized-trial)

Patients were randomly assigned to two groups. The first group was asked to apply sun-protection factor 15+ sunscreen to their face, neck, arms, and hands each morning and after bathing, after spending more than a few hours in the sun, or after sweating heavily. The second group was asked to use sunscreen at their discretion. Participants were also randomly assigned to receive daily beta-carotene or placebo pills. Impressions were taken of the backs of participants' hands at the beginning of the study and 4.5 years later. The impressions were examined for microscopic changes of skin aging by assessors who did not know to which study groups the participants had been assigned.

Researchers found that those in the daily use group were less likely to have increased skin aging after 4.5 years than were those in the discretionary use group. No difference in aging was seen between persons who received beta-carotene pills and those who received placebo pills.

(See further research on: https://www.ncbi.nlm.nih.gov/pubmed/24417448)

Steven Wang, M.D., Director of Dermatologic Surgery and Dermatology, Memorial Sloan Kettering Cancer Center, New Jersey, says wearing sunscreen every day, even when it's cloudy, even when you leave and return from work in the dark, is scientifically proven as the most effective way to preserve and attain a youthful appearance.

Before spending hundreds of dollars on anti-aging products, apply broad-spectrum SPF 30—not just a makeup that has SPF—every single day, without exception. And don't forget your chest and neck.

Conclusion: Daily use of sunscreen seems to protect against skin aging.

Dangerous Moles

Dermatologist Henry Wiley MD advises the earliest and possibly best indicator of possible danger is a change in a mole. A change is any change. Often patients think that change means only darker or bigger or bleeds, but change can also mean lighter, smaller, different shape, different size, a different feeling (like itching), or hair falling out of a mole. If a mole is different in any way, it should be carefully considered for removal. The second major indicator of possible trouble is irregularity in a mole. And a third and strange warning sign of possible cancerous changes in a mole, Dr. Wiley says, is if your dog keeps sniffing the mole. (https://www.drhenrywiley.com/moles, https://www.ncbi.nlm.nih.gov/pmc/articles/PMC2690513/)

If caught early, precancerous moles can be safely and easily removed before they turn into a deadly cancer.

Fight Diabetes

According to the American Diabetes Society, almost 30 million Americans, 9.3% of the population, have diabetes. 86 million Americans have pre-diabetes. 1.7 million Americans are diagnosed with diabetes every year. Age 65 years or older, 11.2 million, or 25.9% of all people in this age group, have diabetes.

Eliminate Toxins

Dr. Joseph Pizzorno N.D., author of *The Toxin Solution,* says toxicity has become the primary driver of disease in the industrial world. Thousands of studies exist showing we have high levels of persistent organic pollutants (POPs), arsenic, cadmium, lead, and mercury, and that they cause disease.

A 2016 study in the *Environmental Health Perspective Journal* suggests that POP, persistent organic pollutant, exposure, including pesticides, heavy metals, solvents, plasticizers, and industrial chemicals, may be the most significant factor for developing diabetes. Obese people who are low in POPs don't appear to have an increased risk of diabetes, as compared with the rest of the population. Instead it appears that obesity combined with elevated POP levels are the most significant risk factors for developing diabetes. Integrative physicians suggest that eliminating stored toxins through a detoxification protocol is key to preventing diabetes and other chronic illnesses. (https://restorativemedicine.org/digest/environmental-medicine-expert-dr-joseph-pizzorno-to-demystify-detoxification/)

Maintain a Healthy Weight

The American Diabetes Society recommends losing weight. Choose healthy foods, make healthy meals, and be active at least thirty minutes a day.

To lose weight, nutritionists recommend eating less. To achieve this, keep an honest record of food you eat for a few days. Eliminate foods with fat, fried food, food high in salt, sweets, baked goods, beverages with added sugar like soda, sports drinks, and energy drinks. Substitute with water or tea. Drink alcohol in moderation. Eat healthy food from all food groups: vegetables, fruits, grains, protein, dairy. Eat small portions.

A Sept 17, 2014 study in the journal *Nature* introduces a new idea: Diet sodas may alter our gut microbes in a way that increases the risk of metabolic diseases such as Type 2 Diabetes in some people. Researchers at the Weizmann Institute of Science in Israel fed zero-calorie sweeteners, including saccharin, aspartame and sucralose, to mice and also, in a subsequent study, to humans. Their experiments show that artificial sweeteners can alter the mix of bacteria in the guts of mice and people in a way that can lead some to become glucose intolerant. (https://www.nature.com/news/sugar-substitutes-linked-to-obesity-1.15938 https://www.weizmann-usa.org/news-media/in-the-news/research-shows-zero-calorie-sweeteners-can-raise-blood-sugar)

      A recent study found that eating a gram of cinnamon, maybe a sprinkle in coffee or on cereal, can cause a drop in blood sugar for people with Type 2 Diabetes. (https://www.npr.org/sections/thesalt/2013/12/30/255778250/cinnamon-can-help-lower-blood-sugar-but-one-variety-may-be-best)

      Physical activity helps insulin get glucose into cells and muscle. The ADS recommends adopting a routine of regular activity such as walking, using the stairs, moving around throughout the day. Also recommended is aerobic exercise, such as brisk walking, swimming, or dancing, and strength training, like lifting light weights and flexibility exercises, such as stretching.

      I first became really aware of diabetes when my mom got a diabetes scare 25+ years after her beating cancer. Her sugar levels became too high and she had to get it under control, and fortunately she did. It prompted me to get my levels checked during a physical and sure enough, my sugar levels were getting high. Not quite in any danger zone, but still enough for concern. I couldn't believe it as I always ate really well, or at least I thought I did. My big mistake was thinking that I burned the massive amount of carbs I ingested during all my extreme physical activities. The other bad assumption I made was that all wheat products and brown rice were unequivocally good for you. Wrong again.

    I cleaned it up by reducing my carbs (including changing from brown rice to hulled barley) and was doing fine until the child of a fellow scientist was diagnosed with full blown Type 1 Diabetes. He did the research and we had a few in-depth meetings where he finally said he would prove it to me that my diet was still marginal by having me test my blood sugar for a week or two. I checked before and after each meal and documented what the meals consisted of and sure enough, my blood sugar spiked wildly from a few items that I thought were acceptable.

    I always thought fruit was good for you, but it turns out all simple carbohydrates convert to sugar. My new strategy is to extremely minimize carbs and save your carb intake for moderate portions of things that are worth it, e.g., I still eat a small portion of dark chocolate, but no more fruit, not even blueberries as ultimately they are all sugar. I also will eat an open face sandwich only on bread that is very high fiber. I also cut my cereal intake in half and focused again on the high fiber All-Bran and ground Golden Brown Flax seeds to make up for the loss of the standard cereals.

 The other change which wasn't that hard was changing to light beer only. No more heavy beers and/or wine. Of course, I still follow the 80/20 rule and eat perfectly 80% of the time so I can splurge when the 20% that is worth it appears in my feed bag vicinity.

 I think the No. 1 deficiency in most people's diets is the lack of emphasis on green vegetables. That is the item that you can and should eat massive amounts of: spinach, broccoli, asparagus, brussel sprouts, collard greens, etc. Try melting a little cheese on any green vegetable and it really hits the spot. I follow the greens with a variety of nuts to get my fill (and get full) without having to resort to the sugars and worthless carbs that are so pervasive in today's food choices and availability.

 The staples of a Mediterranean diet—vegetables, fruits, legumes, whole grains, fish and red wine—are recommended in the fight against diabetes, as is using extra-virgin olive oil in salads and when cooking.

 Even good foods can be bad for you. Pesticides used on the food people eat are a better predictor of Type 2 Diabetes than any other factor we have today, says Dr. Joseph Pizzorno, author of *The Toxin Solution*, the founding president of Bastyr University and the co-author of the *Encyclopedia of Natural Medicine* and *The Clinician's Handbook of Natural Medicine*.

Dr. Pizzorno says people in the top 10 percent of toxic exposure have a 20-fold increase risk for Diabetes. The chemicals are insulin receptor site poisons. So, insulin receptors can't respond because they are being poisoned by those persistent organic pollutants.

Fight Heart Disease

Heart disease is the leading cause of death for people of most ethnicities in the United States, including African Americans, Hispanics, and Whites. For American Indians or Alaska Natives and Asians or Pacific Islanders, heart disease is second only to cancer. About 610,000 people die of heart disease in the United States every year. That's 1 in every 4 deaths.

High blood pressure, high cholesterol and smoking are key risk factors for heart disease. About half of Americans (47%) have at least one of these three risk factors.

Medical conditions and lifestyle choices can also put people at a higher risk for heart disease, including: diabetes, being overweight or obese, poor diet, physical inactivity, and excessive alcohol use.

Hardcore Health: Live Young!

To keep your blood moving through your arteries and to prevent plaque clogging up your arteries, the CDC and the American Heart Association recommend:

Keep your weight in a healthy range.

Avoid saturated fats and trans fats, and avoid foods containing partially hydrogenated vegetable oils. Use oils like olive oil and avocado oil.

Choose low-fat dairy and skinless chicken and fish. Eat less red meat.

Eat small portions.

Limit salt and sugar.

Eat vegetables like avocados, walnuts, garlic, olive oil, omega-3 fatty acids found in fish like wild salmon and ocean trout, omega-7 fatty acids found in macadamia nuts and anchovies, cooked tomatoes or pasta sauce.

Nutrients to protect your heart include antioxidants as found in organic blueberries and dark, green vegetables, and recent super-star PQQ, Pyroloquinoline Quinone, a novel vitamin-like compound found in plant foods and PPQ-rich foods like parsley, green peppers, kiwi fruit, papaya, and green tea.

One alcoholic drink a night for women and up to two for men seems to have a beneficial effect. Avoid excessive alcohol.

Don't smoke and avoid secondhand smoke.

If your doctor agrees, take half a regular aspirin or two baby aspirin a day with a glass of water.

Floss regularly to avoid gum inflammation.

Know your blood pressure numbers, and prevent high blood pressure from developing. (For more information see: https://www.ncbi.nlm.nih.gov/pubmedhealth/PMH0062943/)

Healthy Heart
Lower Blood Pressure

Keep your heart healthy by lowering blood pressure. High blood pressure is a common disease in which blood flows through blood vessels, or arteries, at higher than normal pressures. Blood pressure is the force of blood pushing against the walls of your arteries as the heart pumps blood. High blood pressure, sometimes called hypertension, is when this force against the artery walls is too high. Your doctor may diagnose you with high blood pressure if you have consistently high blood pressure readings.

To manage high blood pressure, doctors recommend healthy eating. Foods that lower blood pressure include:

Leafy greens. Potassium helps your kidneys get rid of more sodium through your urine.

Berries. Berries, especially blueberries, are rich in natural compounds called flavonoids.

Hardcore Health: Live Young!

Red beets
Skim milk and yogurt
Oatmeal
Bananas
Salmon, mackerel, and fish with omega-3s
Seeds
Staying physically active, maintaining a healthy weight, quitting smoking, and managing stress are also recommended by doctors for lowering blood pressure.
https://www.nhlbi.nih.gov/health-topics/high-blood-pressure

Lower Cholesterol

Approximately 13 percent of U.S. adults have high total cholesterol. Lowering cholesterol levels can slow down, reduce, or even stop plaque from building up in the walls of arteries, and may decrease the chance of having a heart attack. Mainstays in treating high cholesterol include diet, weight loss, physical activity, and when necessary, drug treatment.
(https://nccih.nih.gov/health/tips/cholesterol)

Heart Attack:

According to the American Heart Association, most heart attacks start slowly, with mild pain or discomfort. Often people affected aren't sure what's wrong and wait too long before getting help. Here are signs that can mean a heart attack is happening:

Chest discomfort. Most heart attacks involve discomfort in the center of the chest that lasts more than a few minutes, or that goes away and comes back. It can feel like uncomfortable pressure, squeezing, fullness or pain.

Discomfort in other areas of the upper body. Symptoms can include pain or discomfort in one or both arms, in the area between shoulder blades, left shoulder, shoulders, the back, neck, jaw or stomach.

Shortness of breath with or without chest discomfort.

Other signs may include breaking out in a cold sweat, nausea or lightheadedness.

As with men, women's most common heart attack symptom is chest pain or discomfort. But women are somewhat more likely than men to experience some of the other common symptoms, particularly shortness of breath, nausea/vomiting, and back or jaw pain. Learn about the warning signs of heart attack in women. Learn the signs, but remember this: Even if you're not sure it's a heart attack, have it checked out. Minutes matter! Fast action can save lives — maybe your own.

Chew an aspirin if experiencing any symptoms. Don't wait. Call 911.
Warning Signs of a Stroke:

FAST—this is the word to remember if you or someone else thinks they might have suffered a stroke.

> F – Face – Ask the person to smile. Does one side of the face droop?
> A – Arms – Ask the person to lift both arms. Does one arm drift downwards?
> S – Speech – Ask the person to repeat a simple phrase. Is speech slurred or strange?
> T – Time – If you see any of these signs, call 911 immediately. Note the time of the first symptom.

Face drooping on one side, one arm feeling weak or numb, speech difficulty or slurred. Even if symptoms cease, don't wait—call 911 or your emergency response number. Chew an aspirin if you have any of these symptoms and get medical advice.

There are two things you can do immediately if someone has a heart attack that could greatly improve their chances of surviving a heart attack—and you want to do them in this order.

1. Call for an ambulance! Time is of the essence. The first thing you want to do is call for an ambulance and then stay at the person's side until help arrives. If the person is unconscious, call 911 and then begin CPR. If you think you're having a heart attack, call for an ambulance and don't attempt to drive yourself to the emergency room.

2. Next, give the person an aspirin to chew on until the ambulance arrives. Chewing the aspirin (not swallowing it) helps to get it into the bloodstream quicker. You also want to make sure you're giving the person a true aspirin, not ibuprofen, acetaminophen, or another pain reliever. That's because aspirin is a highly effective blood thinner. It's a good idea to keep aspirin on-hand in your purse or wallet, in case you or someone near you suffers a heart attack.

KEY NUTRIENT DEFICIENCIES IN THE U.S.

We can easily see which foods we need to eat more of by studying the foods we are deficient in. The acronym for the Standard American Diet is S.A.D., and sadly it can be. Shockingly, many Americans' diets are deficient in key nutrients. The reasons? Industrial agriculture's push for high yields at the expense of nutrient density, plus our own addiction to eating processed junk. We are overfed and undernourished.

Here is a list of the key nutrients most lacking in the average diet and the percentage of people with a dietary intake below the average requirement. Also included are the naturally occurring sources of the nutrient:

Vitamin D: 95%—Found in fatty fish, mushrooms, sunlight, fortified milk

Vitamin E: 94%—Found in nuts, seeds, green leafy vegetables

Magnesium: 61%—Found in whole grains, wheat bran, leafy green vegetables, legumes

Vitamin A: 51%—Found in liver, fatty fish, milk, eggs, carrots, pumpkins, tomatoes, leafy green vegetables

Calcium: 49%—Found in milk, yogurt, cheese, kale, broccoli

Vitamin C: 43%—Found in all fruits particularly citrus and vegetables, tomatoes

Vitamin B6: 15%—Found in fish, beef, poultry, starchy vegetables

Folate: 13%—Found in spinach, liver, asparagus, brussel sprouts, added to flour

Zinc: 11%—Found in red meat, poultry, beans, nuts

Iron: 8%—Found in meat, seafood, legumes, added to enriched flour

Vitamin B12: 4%—Found in fish, meat, poultry, eggs, milk

Iodine—Found in iodized salt, seafood, seaweed, egg yolks, milk. Iodine deficiency, related to thyroid problems and birth defects is a growing problem worldwide

Dietary intake information from the National Health and Nutrition Examination Survey. https://www.cdc.gov/nchs/nhanes/index.htm

FOODS TO AVOID
Sugar and Soda, Chips and Corn Chips

I have been a strong advocate for avoiding "sugar water" or soda/pop as it is so coyly referred to. When I was a little kid, I saw a demonstration of how much dry white sugar equivalent is in each can of soda. I was shocked, realizing I would never stir that much sugar into anything the size of a can of soda.

Stirring chemical sweeteners into water has its own set of problems. It violates one of my rules when it comes to food: avoid the color white. The food shouldn't be processed and the person preparing it should not have a white coat on!

On the economical side, it never made sense to me to pay for drinks when a better alternative, a glass of water, is free. The only thing I drink besides water is light beer, and almond milk in my cereal.

Many Americans have taken note of the many studies indicating that drinking sodas is bad for their health. Consumption has been steadily decreasing during the past decade, and the downward trend continues. A recent Gallup poll found that 63 percent of people "actively" tried to avoid soda compared to only 41 percent in 2002.

Calories from sugar are more easily turned into fat than calories from other sources. Harvard University found that 12-year-old girls who drank sugary sodas were more likely to be obese than those who avoided them, and, for each additional soda daily, the risk of obesity increased more than

Hardcore Health: Live Young!

150 percent. (https://www.hsph.harvard.edu/nutritionsource/sugary-drinks-fact-sheet/)

Diet sodas may alter our gut microbes in a way that increases the risk of metabolic diseases such as Type 2 Diabetes—at least in some of us. Researchers at the Weizmann Institute of Science in Israel describe what happened when they fed zero-calorie sweeteners, including saccharin, aspartame and sucralose, to mice. To their surprise, the mice developed glucose intolerance. (https://directorsblog.nih.gov/2014/10/07/taking-a-new-look-at-artificial-sweeteners/)

The research team, which included Eran Elinav, an immunologist, and Eran Segal, a computational biologist, examined clinical data from 400 people taking part in an ongoing nutrition study. That analysis found that, compared to people who didn't use artificial sweeteners, long-term users of artificial sweeteners tended to have higher blood glucose levels often associated with diseases like diabetes, obesity, and fatty liver.

The American Heart Association recommends severely limiting foods fried commercially, such as packaged fried tortilla chips, to reduce your risk of developing high cholesterol and high blood pressure.

Weight-loss specialist Charlie Seltzer, MD, says the most scientifically proven way to live longer and feel younger is to maintain a healthy body weight. He adds that this may seem simple, but no amount of antioxidants or vitamins or a super low-calorie diet will make up for carrying extra weight, especially around your belly. (See more at: http://www.drseltzerweightloss.com/)

The Centers for Disease Control and Prevention 2015 report takes a new approach to spur more Americans to take steps to prevent cardiovascular disease, heart attacks, and strokes. Nearly 3 out of 4 U.S. adults have a heart that's older than the rest of their bodies, according to CDC calculations. The report's lead author, CDC scientist Quanhe Yang, says heart disease is the nation's No. 1 killer, but the bottom line is that you can do some very simple things to become younger at heart. (https://www.cdc.gov/heartdisease/)

The CDC recommends maintaining a healthy weight by controlling what you eat, getting enough physical activity, not smoking or using other forms of tobacco, and limiting alcohol use.

A recent analysis from the University of North Carolina at Chapel Hill determined that aspirin's one-two punch outweighs its downsides. They concluded low-dose aspirin can cut your risk for a first heart attack by at least 22 percent while lowering risk for strokes caused by blood clots, and for the leg pain of peripheral artery disease. In contrast, aspirin increases risk for digestive-system bleeding by about 2.5 percent. Ask your doctor about whether daily low-dose aspirin would be

good for you.
(https://www.ncbi.nlm.nih.gov/pubmed/26583574.)

CHAPTER 3— MENTAL

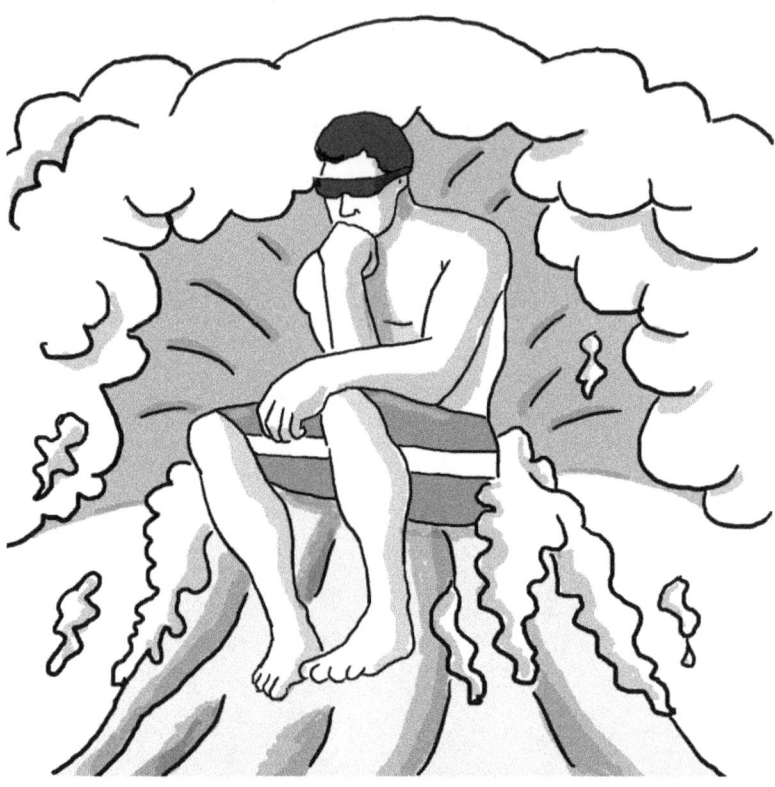

GOALS AND A SENSE OF PURPOSE.
    What do you really want out of your life? What activity, work, career or passion motivates you and gives your life meaning? Let the answer to these questions drive you both physically and mentally. Focus on the goals you set and construct a strategy or road map on how to get there and sustain things once you get there.

Hardcore Health: Live Young!

Don't be afraid to compete and fail. The lessons you learn may get you to a higher, more satisfying goal when you reach it. The road to your goal may be twisted and include a few steps backward for every step forward. Sometimes we learn more from our failures than our successes. They challenge you more, that's for sure. Failure and losing can lead to good stuff if taken constructively. If nothing else, they drive you to try harder.

I like to set incredibly high, almost unattainable goals; that way, even if I get close, I am pretty high up in the stratosphere! Once you get used to failure or disappointment, you become much tougher mentally. A professor told me he would rather have a B student who worked really hard, rather than the straight A student who never had to work hard and also never experienced failure of any kind. Failure defines us, especially as entrepreneurs, if you are so inclined.

Back in my basketball days, I derived much satisfaction from winning a game with a bunch of rag-tag underdog guys playing against some top players. It just feels good to win against the odds. I always seem to root for the underdog, perhaps because I consider myself an underdog in many aspects of life.

Another important concept is to recognize what you are good at and also what you are not good at. Don't try to force something if that is not your strength. On the other hand, always try to improve your areas of weakness in order to become an all-round better person or competitor.

If you keep your overall life road map in the back of your mind, it helps when you encounter setbacks. Too often, people let setbacks defeat them completely. It's strange, but sometimes setbacks propel you in a slightly different direction that turns out to be a better route to achieve your goals.

When you're young, you tend to let the highs be a little too high and the lows a little too low. In other words, try to take all victories and defeats in stride and keep moving (or crawling) forward.

Another thing that I've experienced is that the thrill of victory is even sweeter if you have worked hard for it and/or you achieved it against some mounting odds. Anyone can win when they are not injured and are on the best team. It's the opposite scenario that's really impressive and personally rewarding. Harder is better. Achievement is measured not only in the end result, but also in the path taken to arrive at that goal.

On a more primitive level, it is hard to focus when you are constantly bombarded with external stimuli. I don't know how we as a society arrived at a point where it is acceptable for people to have little televisions in their pockets bombarding them with advertisements and other fluff. For obvious reasons, I choose nature over everything else when it comes to focus. Solitude in nature is, at least for me, the most cleansing thing I can do to bring clarity in any challenge or creative endeavor. Whether it's being in nature or something else like meditating, find a place or an activity that enables you to think clearly and relax and helps you reset your mind, providing a clean slate for what comes next on your life's road map.

BRAIN HEALTH

An analysis in 2017 by a National Academies of Sciences, Engineering and Medicine (NASEM) committee has cited encouraging, although inconclusive, evidence for three specific types of interventions to prevent dementia and cognitive decline with age: cognitive training, blood pressure control for people with hypertension, and increased physical activity.

Cognitive training

Interventions aimed at enhancing reasoning, memory, and speed of processing, to delay or slow age-related cognitive decline were found promising. The committee found no evidence however to suggest that cognitive training might prevent, delay or slow development of Mild Cognitive Impairment (MCI) or Alzheimer's.

Blood pressure management for people with hypertension

Encouraging but inconclusive evidence suggests that blood pressure management, particularly in midlife, might prevent, delay or slow clinical Alzheimer's-type dementia.

Increased physical activity
Citing the many known health benefits of physical activity, the committee pointed to growing evidence that physical activity reduces age-related cognitive decline.
(https://www.nih.gov/news-events/news-releases/national-academies-committee-sees-promising-inconclusive-evidence-interventions-prevent-cognitive-decline-dementia)

What Helps Your Brain:
Exercise, aerobic and strength training, may help your brain stay healthy. Exercising for at least 30 minutes or more a day is recommended.

Staying socially and intellectually active— Read books, write letters, learn a new language, volunteer, play cards, attend worship services, and talk to friends.

A healthy diet— Studies of the Mediterranean Diet justify eating less meat, more nuts, beans, whole grains, salmon, vegetables and olive oil.

Good sleep— Poor sleep quality is linked to Alzheimer's. Several studies found treating sleep apnea helped delay memory problems.

Hardcore Health: Live Young!

What Harms Your Brain?
Depression— In midlife, depression doubles the risk for cognitive decline and dementia, possibly because depression causes changes in the hippocampus of your brain.

Hearing loss— A 2011 study at John Hopkins University found that older adults with hearing problems appear to have a greater rate of brain shrinkage as they age. http://www.chicagotribune.com/lifestyles/health/sc-health-0121-hearing-loss-dementia-20150115-story.html

Certain medications— Drugs like anti-histamines, including Benadryl, and sleep medications, such as Tylenol PM, increase the risk of dementia. Duke University says it is not advising not to take them ever, but to watch out and be aware of the side affects.

Stress
Long term stress is linked to faster rates of decline in brain health. We can't avoid a lot of the stuff the world throws our way, but we can control the way we react to those events.

Ways to Handle Stress:
Live for today. Make the most of the present. Don't dwell on past mistakes or worry about possible future disasters that may never happen.

Cultivate friends who will be there for you in times of stress. Do the same for them.

Sexual activity releases stress and can mend even the bitterest argument with a partner or spouse. Touch and sexual relations stimulate the brain to release the hormone oxytocin, one of the hormones that bind people together.

See a conflict from the other person's point of view.

Let go of resentment.

Don't blame yourself for disappointments, or focus on them; substitute other goals.

Give yourself a time-out. Take a deep breath.

Smile. Watch a comedy. Read a humorous book. Whether you're laughing at a rerun of *Ferris Bueller's Day Off* or giggling at a cartoon, laughter does you good.

The Mayo Clinic says that laughter is a great form of stress relief. Laughter lightens your load mentally and actually induces physical changes in your body. Laughter increases the endorphins that are released by your brain. It also activates and relieves your stress response, causing a good, relaxed feeling. Laughter soothes tension. (https://www.mayoclinic.org/healthy-lifestyle/stress-management/in-depth/stress-relief/art-20044456)

Negative thoughts cause chemical reactions that can affect your body by bringing more stress into your system. Positive thoughts release neuropeptides that help fight stress and improve your immune system. Laughter even helps your body produce its own natural painkillers. It helps you connect with people and helps lessen depression and anxiety. Laughter makes you feel happier.

 Count your blessings.
 Be organized.
 Make a budget and keep to it.
 Take a walk, listen to music, exercise, take a hot bath or massage.

 Barton Goldsmith Ph.D., psychotherapist and author of *100 Ways to Defeat Depression* and other emotionally healing books, has very good advice. He recommends, when you know you are going through a tough time, that you be gentle with yourself, and kind to your mind and body. Although your world cannot always be moving up, it can't be in a constant downward spiral either.

 When you feel like the world is crashing in on you, it probably is, but it's most likely not terminal even if it feels that way. He recommends taking a mental health day and relax in the sun, use your home as a hideaway, read, watch a movie, take a yoga class. Be easy on yourself and do what you need to do to avoid a breakdown and to get back to where you once were. It's never as simple as it sounds, Dr. Goldsmith says, but it is doable.

Air Pollution

Long term exposure to air pollution is linked to brain shrinkage, brain damage, and impaired brain function.

Vitamin D
While vitamin D deficiency has been linked to a decline in brain health, there is no evidence that taking vitamin D supplements improves memory. So look for natural sources of vitamin D such as fatty fish like salmon, mackerel and tuna, lean meats, poultry, beans, eggs, and nuts, and exposure to sunshine.

Keep Your Mind Fit
Reading is taking a big blow with the proliferation of electronic devices and videos, however there may be nothing more effective at keeping your mind fit than reading, from toddler to centurion. My father and grand aging-master has remained incredibly sharp and current at 95 years-of-age by religiously reading the entire newspaper everyday, including the editorial sections where complex issues are argued from all perspectives. I have adopted this technique and find it incredibly powerful. Not only do you stay up on all the news and current events, but you exercise your mind by reading and contemplating the subject matter. You just don't get the depth or cerebral workout from watching the TV news or even reading abbreviated coverage on the internet.

Hardcore Health: Live Young!

UCLA's Dr. Gary Small, co-author of The Healthy Brain Kit, found that a two-week program of mental training can actually rewire the brain. He says he has seen evidence on brain scans that memory improves, and recommends strengthening your mind every day by doing crossword puzzles, Sudoku, or Brain Games, a handheld electronic game developed by Dr. Small, that uses numbers, sequences, and word play to condition the left and right spheres of the brain.

Brain Food

A recent study published in *JMA Internal Medicine* found that supplementing the already brain-healthy Mediterranean diet with additional servings of nuts and olive oil enhances memory and information processing. The unsaturated fats in nuts, particularly walnuts, work deep in the brain to fight inflammation and amyloid plaques. (https://jamanetwork.com/journals/jamainternalmedicine/fullarticle/2293082)

Majid Foruhi, M.D., Medical Director of Neuro Grow Brain Fitness Center and affiliate staff at John Hopkins Medicine in Baltimore, says following the Mediterranean diet for six months will sharpen your brain. The supplemented diet makes your brain less susceptible to Alzheimer's disease decades later.

Other foods Dr. Foruhi recommends to help brain health are fish, blueberries, grapes, and dark chocolate. (http://neurogrow.com/)

POSITIVE PESSIMISM (A FORM OF OPTIMISM)

Expect the worse and whatever you get is better than you expected. I have tried to live my life by this mantra. It helps smooth out the highs and lows of life and more specifically prepares you for the negative things that occur. I still consider myself an optimist, however I like to hedge those bets by remaining prepared for the worst. Essentially, it is a survival technique that fits my professional career of developing survival technology and procedures.

There is a hierarchy of negative things. One of my favorite quotes is from Woody Allen, where he talks about the "horrible and the miserable." Woody says that someone with cancer or paralysis is in the category of "horrible" and the rest of us are just "miserable." So you should be thankful, he says, if you're miserable, because that's very lucky, to be miserable. Of course it's a joke, however it puts things into perspective!

When you're confronted with something that is in the horrible category, that doesn't mean it is a life (or death) sentence. A family member of mine was diagnosed with stage 4 cancer, however through chemotherapy, diet adjustment, and mental visualization, she has been able to beat that cancer and remain in remission for over 25 years! When faced with your own mortality, you can either quit or fight.

The "will to survive" also speaks to the mental capacity people have to survive horrible situations. See Louie Zamperini's story in *Unbroken.* Louie spent 47 days lost at sea in a raft followed by two years of torture in a POW camp. Another hero of mine is General William Spruance, an aviator horribly injured in a plane crash who was able to survive and share his experience and philosophies well into his 90's (including sewing his arm into an opening in his stomach for months to aid in the healing of his burns)!

Positive pessimism enables me to assume there are cancer cells in my body engaged in battle with my immune system, however I remain confident that I can beat them down by always staying in top shape on all fronts.

BALANCE

Try to keep a healthy mix of work, play and training in both the physical and mental sectors. If you constantly think of work only, it's hard to let your mind take a breather. When you're working, try to attack problems with your mind that may not necessarily be your responsibility. I like to occasionally brainstorm and try to solve mega-problems that may be unsolvable. Just by leaving your daily grind of work problems even for a few minutes and then returning to them can provide a much needed break for your mind.

We have already discussed the various aspects of recreation and training that can be tailored to your own interests. Cross-training is a powerful process that has become popular recently because it makes a lot of sense. Try to use all parts of your body and mind because ultimately they are all connected. It gives you a chance to rest certain sectors of your mind on auto-pilot while you are focusing heavily on another process.

Years ago, I had some friends who were making fun of some of my colleagues for their passion for stupid slapstick comedy. They couldn't understand why such intelligent people could find what they considered fluffy comedy so entertaining. I guess they were snobs. However the more I thought about it, the more convinced I was that highly intelligent people like to give their minds a rest and keep it balanced with a healthy dose of mindless entertainment. There is nothing like a good laughing session, no matter where you obtain the source material (as long as it is not hurtful to others).

Over the years, I have performed a lot of outreach education to students of all ages. The one thing that cuts across all ages is the fact that, if they are laughing, they are learning. They are much more engaged if they are happy or amused by portions of the material or presentation. It seems like their intake valves are wide open once you trigger that laughter button.

Studies also show that when students are working on a real-life project, they are way more engaged and learn and retain much more of the reading/writing/arithmetic that is intrinsic to the overall project than if they were just required to sit and listen to a dry set of lectures on the subject. I believe this is another good example of the value of keeping things balanced.

TAKE A BREAK

On a practical level, we all need to take breaks during our normal work schedule. I've found if you mix these breaks with your daily requirements you can optimize your day and keep your mind balanced. For example, if I need to take a work break I combine it with an errand I have to run at the bank and facilitate with a bike for transportation. Therefore, I get the work break, complete the errand, and get a little physical work out and fresh air.

I think this is one of the most powerful things people can do to improve their physical shape. Don't work out just to work out. Run errands by walking or biking, that way forcing yourself to get some exercise during a required task. If you live or work in a city, an easy way to accomplish this is to never use the elevator, always use the stairs. If you live in the suburbs and it is too far to walk or bike to the bank, make sure you park your car at the furthest point from the store in the parking lot, and then walk briskly to and from the store, as well as within the store. Once again, you will have earned the completion of that errand. It feels good, as all little accomplishments do!

On a larger scale, I have an idea that I believe will help solve the country's obesity problem and other health care issues: Food Towers. Hire the best healthy chefs you can and have them cook incredible healthy meals and provide it for free (subsidized by the government and private advertisers). The only catch is that the meals are served 10+ stories up and you have to walk. You are only allowed to stay up there for 45 minutes and then you have to walk back down. The stairwells could have defibrillators in case people keel over and there could be advertisements throughout to subsidize the costs.

One thing is for sure, people respond to free stuff and this is a way to essentially trick them into getting exercise and eating healthy. Of course it would be completely voluntary and it could even be located next to your favorite fast food restaurant. That would go a long way to solving a bunch of health care issues in this country (and increasingly, the world). Although it sounds like a joke, it is 90% serious. Perhaps a wealthy philanthropist will take me up on the idea and begin to open Food Towers in abandoned buildings?

The concept of taking breaks and earning your food or money makes a lot of sense to me as an avid observer of nature. This is how it's done in nature. Animals hunt or gather (i.e., they earn it) and then take breaks and recharge their batteries before they repeat the process.

It has become way too easy for modern humans to get their food without earning it, not to mention the low quality of food they receive by not earning it. Yes, I understand they are exchanging this food for money they earned, however it is obvious to me you should still have a physical expenditure to earn a meal (or at least an intense mental expenditure).

My Push Button Super Fuel main feast described previously is self-awarded after I have completed my two mile paddle break. That way, I feel as though I have earned this bountiful feast. In fact, I often match my quality and quantity of any one meal to the amount of physical (or mental) exertion that I expended prior to that meal. Even in the surf world, if the waves were small and I didn't do so well, I only eat a moderate meal afterwards. If, on the other hand, the waves were huge and death defying and I survived, then of course a feast is in order! Earn it!

REWARD YOURSELF

Rewarding yourself should not be limited to the type and quantities of food you can devour, although that is the reward opportunity that seems to present itself the most (at least three times a day)! A reward can be found in a variety of sectors. After I complete a lot of fruitful work, I try to take a few hours off and watch a movie. maybe even in the middle of the day if I am feeling wild! Let your brain be rewarded as much as your stomach, again with the theme of "earning it." For me, there is no better feeling than indulging yourself with a treat that matches the effort and achievement you just put out. Not only is it gratifying for you in the moment, but it provides fuel for you to go out and strive for your next mini (or massive) achievement.

      It is also very useful to break your life down into smaller segments where you can see the beginning and end of any task. There are, of course, your long-term goals and you can reward those when appropriate; however, if you only award yourself for those, you can get bogged down into thinking you are not progressing fast enough. I think it is analogous to going to sleep at night, another reward that should be fully earned that day. I know that when I finally go to sleep at night, the day has been absolutely packed with tasks and mini-rewards that make me proud of my accomplishments for that day. Sleep recharges me for the next day in the same way that taking a day off and eating bon-bons in bed while binging movies can be completely reinvigorating (and a great guilty pleasure)!

Reward Yourself to Foster Good Habits

To break bad habits, each time you reject a bad habit, reward yourself. When you follow through on what could be a good habit, reward yourself again.

Dr. Oz, author of *You: Staying Young,* says that the boost of dopamine you get from the reward, which can be minor but is something that pleases you, teaches your brain to choose the good habit.

CHAPTER 4—SOCIAL

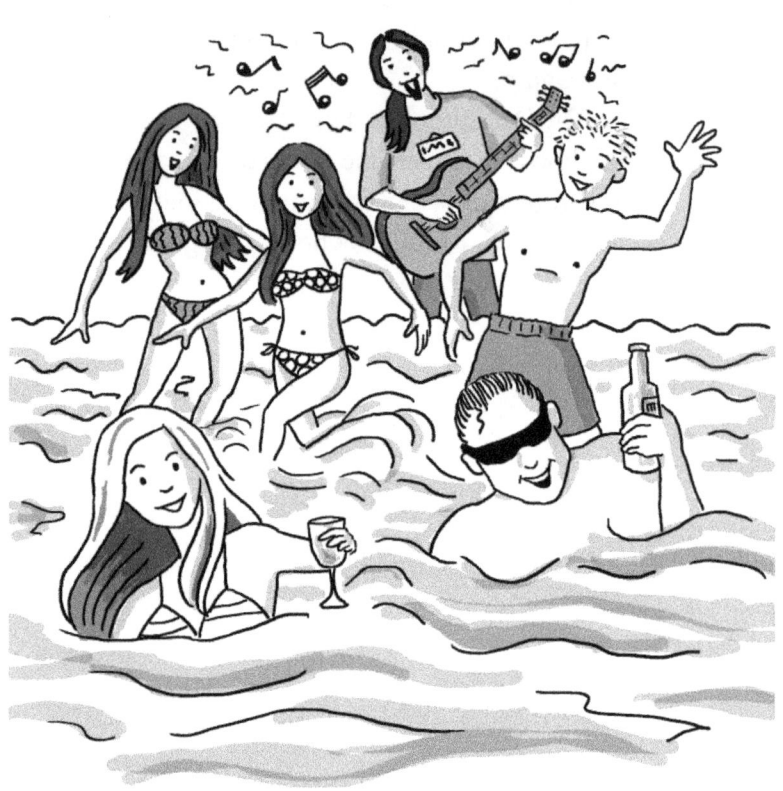

FAMILY

Family for me is the ultimate priority. But remember, you have to take care of yourself first, so you can take care of and provide for everyone else. That is why on the airlines, the FAA instructions tell you to put your oxygen mask on first in the case of an emergency and THEN put them on your children. If you fumble around putting someone else's mask on first, you might pass out and then you all are in trouble.

Family, of course, is a broad term and can be many things to many people. Your family may be a traditional one with a spouse and a few kids or it could be you and your pets. Whatever it is, it is a critical resource to help you live a long and rich life.

From a primitive perspective, that is our main purpose on the planet—to procreate. Anyone who has children knows that pleasure you get from looking into your children's eyes and watching them grow to become adults, even if they are often pains in the ass. There are definitely pros and cons with having children, but fortunately the pros outweighs the cons for most of us.

KIDS

It's not that having children adds to your anti-aging regiment but rather that dealing with them effectively can prevent you from the ultimate aging act, i.e., dying! The stress of raising children is massive, especially dealing with the different stages of their development—a monumental task. On one hand, children keep you active by just trying to keep up with them physically, mentally and emotionally. The larger problem for efficient aging is not letting them get to you and eat away at your core health.

One piece of advice I received prior to having children (while my wife was expecting) was to make the kids fit into your schedule and not the other way around. We took that to heart and took our kids along on the fun things we were doing, including hiking, water sports and even travel. Although some people would argue the point, I believe my mental health has remained intact because of this very practice. Kids are not the center of the universe; the parents are! Kids need to aspire to become adults and not be revered, as they commonly are in these over-indulged times.

It is not easy raising children, but it is extremely rewarding in a similar manner to achieving any major long term goal. A discouraging development, from my perspective, is the way young children and their needs are put at the apex of the family. That is absolutely backwards as children are little interns that have to earn adulthood and that is accomplished by observing (as semi-second class citizens) their parents go about their lives as the leaders of the family. Adult time is something they need to aspire to, not be gifted to right out of the box.

One of the most important things young parents can do is establish the line between adults and children, starting with a fixed baby-sitter date night every weekend so the children can see the adults have their own life and their relationship as the apex, not the kids' needs and desires. Children are smart and will accept this situation or, alternatively, they will work their parents for everything they can get if they see an opening. Establish the hierarchy as soon as possible and let the kids earn it.

If you do your homework early while the kids are young, you will be rewarded later when your well-adjusted young adult children make your advanced aging years less stressful. Maybe, in future years, they can even help you out a little as payback!

FRIENDS AND CLUBS

Human interaction is another key factor for long term health and, although I consider myself a lone wolf, I enjoy interacting with other humans. Developing interactive skills, especially listening, is very important for having fulfilling relationships. If you live in an isolated setting or don't enjoy hanging out with people in your immediate arena, join clubs or other groups with like-minded people with whom you have something in common.

Dan Buettner, author of *The Blue Zones, Eating and Living Like the World's Healthiest People*, found that who you hang out with trumps just about everything else when it comes to health. He says people who live longest surround themselves with people who support healthy behaviors. Buettner introduced the concept of health-conscious communities into the U.S. by forming Blue Zone cities that encourage healthy active living where people hike, plant community gardens, hold vegetable potlucks, and travel together. (See www.bluezones.com.)

It's interesting that whenever people have real trouble in their life, whether it's drugs or traumatic experiences, one of the required rehabilitation efforts centers around getting together with groups of people that have experienced similar things to compare notes and to heal together (e.g., AA, NA, group therapy, etc.). It seems a little backwards that we wait until we are in dire need of this type of interaction before we seek it out or are court-ordered to attend. Rather than waiting, it seems to make more sense to focus on getting involved with groups of people with whom we have similar interests and share our experiences and learn from each other.

These groups can be small, informal ones where you just get together with a few friends (book clubs) or larger organized formal ones (hiking/walking clubs). I've been very fortunate to be part of a large global group of surfers. We commune with each other and compare notes in the ocean in between waves, with the subject matter varying widely from waves to family to politics to jokes to inventions, all in between scurrying around to survive the dynamic ocean.

Often, the process of growing older can isolate us from each other. Taking classes, particularly at local community colleges, can bring us into contact with all sorts of interesting people. In this way, going back to school—the sheer act of going—can invigorate a life by coming together with like-minded others. Did you know that taking a class in just about any subject can improve your cognitive abilities, rejuvenate your memory, grow new brain cells, and be fun all at the same time? Recent scientific studies clearly show that senior citizens who stay mentally active enjoy all of these rewards.

Many states offer free classes or allow seniors to attend (audit) regular classes for free. Discuss your needs and goals with the admissions department of the institution you desire to attend. (See http://www.seniorresource.com/senioreducation.htm for state-by-state educational opportunities for seniors.)

It's very beneficial to have a network of friends on many different levels, from acquaintances to best friends. There is nothing like a good friend and, typically, you can count your good friends on one hand. Commonly, you grew up with them and you have a rapport that is unmatched even by your spouse. They know you better than anyone and they are willing to give you the straight truth on whatever is going on (at least a good friend will). Even just a long distance phone call to a long-lost buddy can provide a great break in your life. It also lets you review past historical feelings and events that can keep you focused on your overall life map and goal.

A friend of mine meets her two sisters regularly for coffee via Skype. She says that they live in three different states and were getting in touch less and less. When they first starting Skype coffee meetings, they had very little to say to one another as they hadn't kept regularly in touch. Now, she says, they talk animatedly about all the little day-to-day things in their lives and it's great.

From a competitive perspective, which I have trouble ignoring, it's also good to check on your old buddies to see how they are doing— especially compared to your own condition in life. I personally derive incentive from talking or hearing of my friends' great accomplishments. First and foremost I am happy for them, but a close second is a nice kick in the ass to get my own act in motion. I think friendly competition is good even if it is all under the surface.

I like to try to maintain layers of friends from various sectors of my life— chronological, geographical and intellectual. Friends from different parts of your life can trigger different thoughts in your mind and bring you back to a place and time or way of thinking that you may have abandoned or at least forgotten about. Friends provide perspective and force you to perform some introspection, which at times can be painful, yet useful.

Hardcore Health: Live Young!

I have always been intrigued by the perceived difference in what people consider success. Growing up, me and my buddies idolized the people who had the best lifestyle— not the most money. On the fringe of the 60's, having a lot of money and material things did not rank as high as they do now. There were no reality stars, idolized for their material goods. It was just the opposite, as we idolized guys living off the land in some distant place, surfing and exploring as a loner or with a small crew of friends and/or tight family.

The other nice thing about keeping a close group of friends is that it forces you to interact on a human basis (and I don't mean Facebook friends). When I connect with a friend, there is a clear pecking order for me on how to go about it: First, and by far the best, is face to face meeting and interaction. Second, is the good old phone call when you actually push the buttons and talk to another human on the other end. A distant third option, is the one-way e-mail or text, but it's hard to gauge a person's reactions with these. If talking face-to-face, you can alter your thoughts in mid-sentence based on the body language of the person you are interacting with. I also subscribe to this pecking order for my work, as it is easy to be misunderstood when you are sending one-way communications back and forth with no body language or voice cues to draw from.

Friends can also include acquaintances who you run into on a daily basis. There is something invigorating about being on the receiving end of a nice smile, especially if you can return the favor and it comes from someone who is part of your daily routine. It gives you a sense of place and belonging, a very healthy interaction that probably compares with the feeling a person gets from being greeted by their spouse on their arrival home.

And maybe smiling is good for you. Jeanne Louis Calmart, who lived 122 years and 164 days, the Guinness World Record, thought so. Calmart rode her bike at 100 years of age and lived on her own till 110, and at 121 released CD's with her musings set to rap, techno and regional music. "Smile," Calmart said. "Always keep your smile. That's how I explain my long life."

Meet like-minded people at health and fitness centers, community college classes, dance classes, movie or theatre groups, hobby clubs, church, book clubs and political groups. Volunteer to help others, teach or share your knowledge at small business centers, coach a youth team, join a park restoration group etc.

Pets are another great source of (quasi) friends. There is nothing like a pet, as they are always there for you and seem to put the world in perspective since they are not a part of the human rat race and are just looking for some food, love and attention. I highly recommend as many pets as possible, not only to force you to walk the neighborhood, but also to have silent friends surrounding you. Of course, if you take this too far, you could become shunned by the rest of humanity, so limit the total amount of animals—unless you live on a farm.

HUMAN INTERACTION AND THE SMARTPHONE

To make real friends, the first step is to turn off those "smart" phones (dumb phones). Everyone seems to be virtually holding hands with their device to make up for the fact they are really alone in their little rooms. Turn off those devices that Steve Jobs tricked you into mainlining like heroin and go outside. Meet a person. Talk to a person. Get lost. Look at nature. Try a new place to eat without being told how good it is. Learn how to look someone in the eye. Experiment with a handshake and even a real two-way, in-person conversation. Social media is really anti-social media, (likely) lulling you into deep isolation, jealousy and depression.

It really bothers me what is going on with the explosion of people (especially kids who have the most to lose) suckling their devices like pacifiers—getting dumber, more socially awkward and less creative with every second. We have to break this cycle and it will not be easy as big money has got a hold of revolving charges—the ultimate scam. The smartest people around are brainstorming new ways to get people more excited and addicted to coming back to their "app" and paying their revolving charges or subjecting themselves to constant advertising bombardment—all the while giving up their privacy as they pinpoint and literally tell you what to do next.

I remember reading *1984* back in the 1970's—that is a walk in the park compared to what's going on now. At least in *1984,* people protested as they were led to slaughter, but that's not so for the people now who anxiously wait in line for the latest phone version to launch. We need to try to get back to real non-virtual stuff, starting with turning off the devices and doing something new—like going outside and talking to a real person (in person)! This works for kids too. Kids build important social skills from these real interactions, as opposed to the virtual world of the "smart" phone.

SOLITUDE

On the other hand, your best friend and the person you can rely on the most is yourself. I am a strong believer in self-reliance a la Emerson and Thoreau with a little mix of *Old Man in the Sea* and *MacGyver.* Learn to be with yourself, alone and in nature. Teach yourself to be comfortable alone with your thoughts and able to survive in any and all situations, whether humans are involved or not. It's funny, but I can find solitude in the most crowded places or in the most remote places. One good place to practice this is on an airplane where you are crammed next to people in a metal tube. I find myself deep in my thoughts for the most part, especially once I put on the noise canceling headphones and shut my eyes.

Take care of yourself first—life is all about survival and thriving; after all, for the most part, no one is taking care of you but you. If you are at peace with yourself, everything else is easy. Practice being alone, deep in nature and deep in public, or eat out alone with a book/newspaper or even more challenging without a book, newspaper or even cell phone!.

Being alone and at peace in your settings, regardless of their complexity or lack thereof, builds confidence. The trick is to not be viewed as a crazy person when alone in public—that is where something to read usually comes in handy.

You also learn to make the best of the situation/location you are in. There is a classic line in *Fast Times at Ridgemont High*, where the older guy is trying to instill confidence in the younger guy about his upcoming date, and states that you have to have "the attitude" that includes the line, "wherever you are, it's the place to be!" You have to make the best of situations and conditions and try to take a positive outlook. Sometimes it takes a creative eye to see the best of your situation or even some slight tweaking to make a bad situation better.

CHAPTER 5—SPIRITUAL

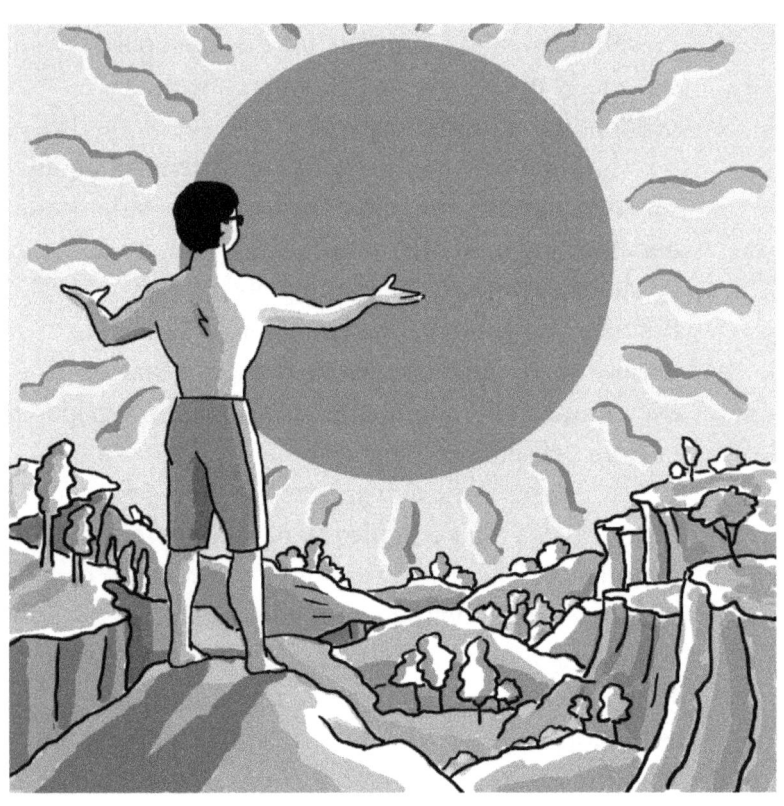

NATURE

Spirituality is a very diverse and personal issue. For me, nature is where I make my deep spiritual connections. I just feel the most connected when I am furthest off the grid, hanging with the other living things, flora and fauna. It's hard to even put into words the feeling of calmness, complacency and content I experience when alone and deep with the creatures.

As a scientist and inventor, I have an endless fascination with observing how natural things work and how living things have evolved in their own specific manner to survive their surroundings. Living things have been around for billions of years, humans only thousands of years, and me, personally, only tens of years— so I humbly take my place on the sidelines and observe the masters.

I also enjoy the simplicity that seems to exist within these highly complex and evolved creatures. It's mostly about where they are getting their next meal—just like us! And you can be sure that they earn it every time!

MUSIC

In nature there are various sounds and rhythms that serve as the background of life. I think humans have recognized this and have riffed on this for years and use music as a way to express the many moods and feelings we all experience.

Music has always been a driving force for me on many levels. Growing up, rock and roll provided the escape and anti-establishment needed at the time. There is just something that completely fires up the physical, mental, emotional and spiritual when a song connects with you. Again, it's hard to describe, but I am sure most people can relate to it.

I enjoy all types of music and like to match the music to the energy level that I am at or want to get to. For instance, I love to listen to classical music when I am problem-solving/creating. For manual labor, I prefer loud rock and roll. For pre-surfing amp up, I also like rock and roll with variations in speed (a little bit of punk/ska). For relaxing, reggae or jazz do the trick. I think we all have internal music clocks that match the external music we expose them to (assuming you are open to it and your clock can handle the settings).

I see music in a similar category to pets as they can change your mood within seconds—a powerful trick! When you feel a little down or lazy, look for the closest dog, cat, or song.

RELIGION

Personal, private and whatever works for you—religion is and can be a powerful grounding force for many people. As long as it works for you, go for it. There are great lessons and road maps in all religions. It's just unfortunate that religion ends up pulling humans apart for lack of respect, even though most religions essentially follow the same principles.

Religion can also be observed equally as well on a private/personal basis as opposed to established organizational functions. Ultimately, it is and should remain a personal choice that can help you. if you so choose, throughout many aspects and stages of life.

SERVICE AND GIVING BACK

A few years ago, during a family medical situation, a friend of mine told me I needed to "lose self" and essentially focus on helping those who needed my help. It was sage advice that I still follow today. Once you have your own situation in order personally, there is nothing more gratifying than helping others who need it more than you.

By losing self, you can focus on the challenge others have, making you appreciate even more what you have. It feels so good to help people, that it has to be good for your overall health, even though that is not the motivation for doing it, but rather a nice fringe benefit.

PART TWO—LIVING CLOSE TO NATURE

INTRODUCTION

In our daily lives, we are constantly faced with challenges, many of which can become great burdens. We simply don't have the time to go out in nature or find the resources to eat healthy. We simply don't make the time necessary to keep in balance our body, mind and spirit. Often, however, it is these challenges that bring about our greatness and these obstacles that bring about our strengths. I want to talk about some of the simpler ways that we can find ourselves getting back to the way of life best for our earth, our loved ones and ourselves.

I moved to the Big Island of Hawaii in the beginning of the New Year 2013. My life as a farmer began as I planted myself on ten acres of land on the beautiful Hāmākua Coast. Deep rich soil and sunny days, mixed with the perfect amount of rain, means one of the most ideal climates for growing most all types of fruit and vegetables. Of course, the land was formerly planted with sugarcane and was at that time growing acres of ten foot high guinea grass, but that is another hard work story.

I danced around the outskirts of true healthy living for years, but found it both difficult and costly. I realized the only way to get around this would be to grow my own organic produce. After a few unsuccessful attempts, I decided to approach

Hardcore Health: Live Young!

the concept of farming by studying Permaculture Design with Geoff Lawton of the Permaculture Institute of Australia. This was a sobering and rewarding exercise. Farming was a scientific field and I had a lot to implement. One of the most important things was starting from scratch with the soil.

By bringing true health to the soil, I could bring true health to myself and my family. This became my mission—to produce the most nutritionally rich food in the land. Only then could I bypass the industrial mayhem occurring in our food supply. The fact that people densely cluster into cities makes for the necessity of factory farms and earth-pillaging farms of agriculture. It seems as if we got something right when you look at the bright shiny conventional produce, but it is really a shiny shell on the outside of a pulp of nutrition-stripped hybrids. These forms of produce are grown on soil poisoned and stripped of all living organisms and force-fed chemicals till they bulk up enough.

As reported by *Scientific American 14* back in 2011, agricultural chemicals destroy the health of the soil by killing off its microbial inhabitants, which is one of the primary problems with modern farming, and the reason why the nutritional quality of conventionally-grown foods is deteriorating. (Read more at: http://homeandgardenamerica.com/organic-food-proven-healthier)

Those who have tasted a homegrown tomato know very well that it blows away all store bought. This is because it is a fruit that gets naturally to its true flavor and ripeness. It harnesses the life force of the microbes in the soil health, and the health benefits of the sun and rain. It is given a chance to become what it truly was made to be. The most powerful foods for health are those that are freshly picked and consumed in their natural raw state— foods such as sprouts, baby greens, juicy fruits, and fresh vegetables. These foods, with their detoxifying, free-radical scavenging properties, have the potential to raise our immunity and energy levels.

Dr. Hans Eppinger, Chief Medical Director at the University of Vienna, found that a live-food diet specifically raised the micro-electrical potential throughout the body. In essence, by restoring the electrical potential of the cells, raw foods rejuvenate the life force and health of the organism. A live-food diet is a powerful natural healing tool in the quest to live young and healthy. (Read more about the energy of live foods at: http://www.yogadream.net/assets/img/pdf/Nutrition/Energy-Live.pdf)

Foods grown with pesticides and herbicides contain a lower life 'pulse' as the soil they are grown in is often depleted of vital nutrients. Organic foods and superfoods are the best way to ensure you receive the most potent life force energy.

Hardcore Health: Live Young!

Eating raw when possible and implementing practices such as lightly steaming versus frying vegetables will ensure your food retains as much of the vital essences as possible.

I've found the best way to bring health to the body is by sustaining a diet of living foods, grass-fed beef, wild caught fish, organic free range chicken, structured water, superfoods and healthy herbs and spices, moderation in grains, dairy and eggs—and moving enough to keep it working.

Adam Crowe, Permaculture Designer and Consultant, Organic Farmer
http://ainaexotics.com/

CHAPTER 6—WE ARE WHAT WE BREATHE, DRINK AND EAT

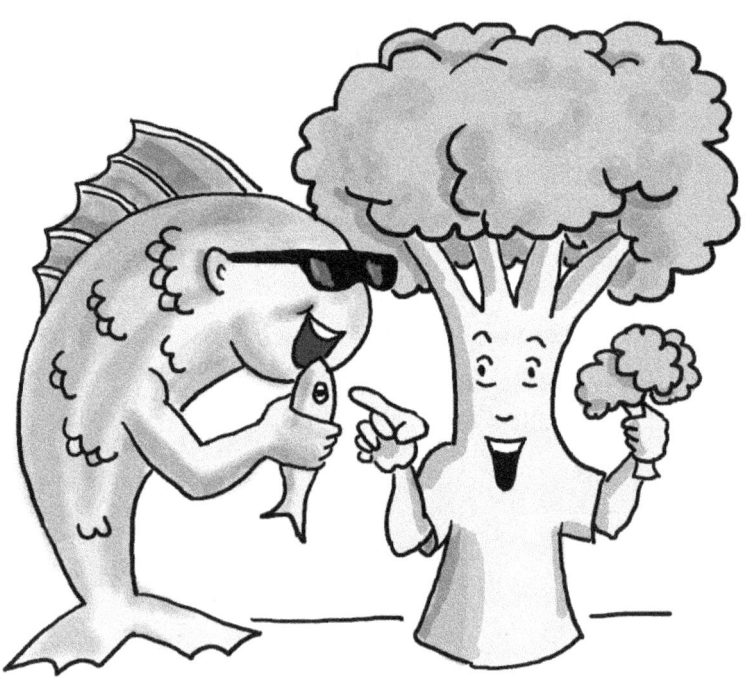

PRIMARY ELEMENTS; AIR, WATER, FIRE AND EARTH

It doesn't take a scientist to see why cancer, inflammatory disease, mental illness, birth defects and obesity are rampant in our society. We are neglecting the primary elements—Air, Water, Fire, Earth—that give us life and trading them for something far less wholesome. This impacts our health. We are what we breathe, drink and eat.

We breathe polluted air in cities, process stale air in our homes, mold and chemicals from drywall, VOC gas from flooring, walls, electronics and insulation, and a host of other issues like black mold, dust and positive ions.

Our water is chlorinated, fluoridated, polluted with chemicals like antidepressants, hormones, rust, lead, arsenic etc. and filtered of all beneficial minerals.

We sit idly in front of the blue light of computers and smartphones or the screens of TV's for an average of 8 hours a day and often face long sunless days in an office, starving ourselves of photonic energy and vitamin D.

We eat foods that are processed, produced with chemical fertilizers and pesticides in depleted soil, low in minerals and vitamins, hybridized to sterility and produced out of season, harvested under-ripe and ripened with chemicals before being treated with fungicide etc.

It is obvious that we have come to neglect the earth's elemental gifts to us. We have shelved the healing elements of the natural order and replaced them with our own version. Only now in the growing generation are we seeing the grave implications of this artificial world we have made within our natural earth.

Fortunately it is very easy to change back. We just have to remember to use our bodies the way nature intends. Like all the other creatures on earth, we need to draw off these elements to survive and sustain ourselves. Without them, our vessels break down.

Air

Air in our homes is toxic often because of VOCs (volatile organic compounds) and gases. Electronics and computers release EMFs (electrical magnetic frequencies). Home insulation is filled with formaldehyde, floors are glued with adhesives and drywall is filled with carcinogens. Make sure your home is ventilated often by opening windows and letting air pass through the house.

Other ways to freshen the air include house plants that are able to absorb VOCs and remove them from the air. Houseplants also help reduce trace amounts of indoor pollutants like formaldehyde (found in new carpeting) and benzene (found in cigarette smoke).

Houseplants recommended by NASA Research scientist Bill Wolverton are:

Areca Palm, Lady Palm, Bamboo Palm, Rubber Plant, Dracaena (especially "Janet Craig"), English Ivy, Dwarf Date Palm, Ficus Alii, Boston Fern and Peace Lily.

Dr. Wolverton also comments that you need a lot of plants to be really effective. He recommends placing a large beautiful plant near your computer and another near your TV, where you spend a lot of time sitting.

Many use air purifiers and filters, but these alone will not remove all contaminant VOCs. They do, however, remove particle matter, like dust, and that can be beneficial to health. A HEPA filter can remove a ton of dust.

Many houses have problems with mold. Burning firewood is one way to dry out the atmosphere. A dehumidifier could greatly benefit a person with a lot of common colds and dampness issues. On the other hand, if you have dry flaky skin, chapped lips and dryness, you would benefit from having house plants, misters, boiling pots of water, or a humidifier unit.

Negative ions can be found in the air where the waves are crashing, where water is hitting stones, at waterfalls and thunderstorms. Negative ion generators are able to cancel out positive ion pollutants. They add electrons to the air and in the process refresh our home atmosphere. Heaven Fresh is a good brand of negative ion generator.

Air conditioner filters should be replaced yearly and air ducts cleaned every three years. Open windows when you can. The quality of air indoors plummets when homes are airtight and the fresh air smell comes from chemicals and chemical fragrance and not actual fresh air.

Take a tip from many Asian nations and leave your shoes, and whatever you might have stepped in, at the front door. Wash your hands as soon as you return to your home.

We are surrounded by chemicals, fire retardants, synthetic materials, pesticides, perfumes, personal care products, make-up, paint and things our bodies are not evolved to deal with. Dr. Joseph Pizzorno, author of *The Toxin Solution* and *The Encyclopedia of Natural Health*, estimates 13.6% of diabetes can be attributed to Diphenyl A, BPA, the synthetic plasticizer found in the lining of canned foods, and 50% of ADHD is attributable to fire retardants, particularly in children's clothing and PCBs, found in plastics, as lubricants and dielectric fluids in transformers, in protective coating for wood, metal and concrete, adhesives, etc.

To help your body fight these toxins, choose organic foods, natural health and beauty products, air new mattresses and furniture and dry cleaned clothes, avoid Teflon-coated cookware

Water

One of the greatest mysteries on our planet is water. We are 50 - 75% water, and everything around us is partly dependent on this element. It is safe to say that water is one thing we all have in common. This also means that water connects us and is constantly affecting us and our energies. We need to take a closer look at this mysterious element and how it can lead us back to our origins and restore our health.

Civilization developed around natural springs and artesian wells. More often than not, any town that has the word "spring" in its name was historically centered around a water flow bubbling up to the surface of the earth. This water would be the basis of setting up life in an area. Many times these springs lost their year-round flow as more and more wells were dug to carelessly irrigate. Many times they simply dried up due to intensive logging or through processes like blowing up headwaters with dynamite to increase water flow. Today, very little awareness exists of one of the most important aspects of human life—the natural spring.

It is no coincidence that springs have been revered for centuries for their healing abilities. You can still find hot-spring resorts that provide therapeutic relief for a variety of afflictions. Many mineral waters bottled throughout the world and sold for a premium price never make it into the hands of many of those who probably need those minerals. In truth, the waters that are bottled are mostly stripped of all beneficial nutrients and left to sit in their plastic bottle accumulating dioxins and bisphenols. In general, most people are led to believe that drinking from springs could be dangerous to your health due to threats like leptospirosis and giardia.

The possibility of contaminants in water has led to state water supply privatizing and capping nearly all of our spring water sources and shrouding their locations in mystery. Any and all springs that are part of the municipal water source are treated with heavy doses of chlorine and other bacteria-killing toxins. The truth is, spring water from true springs, and not a seepage spring, is quite safe to drink but it is better to check with a local who drinks it. Many times you'll see people lined up to get spring water and then you know it's good!

I have visited at least thirty different natural springs around the world and have always found them to be in beautiful locations and the water to be tasty and refreshing with no ill effect whatsoever. Even if you don't find the spring, you usually find a welcoming forest or beautiful neighborhood and mountainside. I've met many kind people at springs, people seeking a higher state of being, and other times people who just know it's damn good water and free like it is supposed to be.

These water sources are often a simple pipe installed by a local resident that makes it possible to fill up jugs by the roadside. More than likely, the spring provides year-round, crystal-clear, pure water. You can gather this water in 5 gallon jugs (BPA Free plastic or glass carboys available at brewing supply stores).

This water will provide intense hydration, flushing toxins and supplementing minerals often deficient from our diets. Most springs are birthed at the same temperature across the world. Meaning, if it's hot out, the spring is still quite cool all year, and in places where it is often freezing temperatures springs will flow at up to 60F year round. In some areas like Thousand Springs Park in Idaho, people use this to their advantage and dive in the spring-fed pools in winter. Check www.findaspring.com for a spring near you.

    It is wise to use a water filter on your faucet or use BPA free jugs at a water machine. However, distilled and reverse osmosis waters are missing key minerals that spring water delivers. If you don't have any natural springs nearby, I recommend adding a pinch of Celtic sea salt to your water to supply minerals and electrolytes that have been removed through filtering.

    Some of the healthiest people I know don't follow all the health rules but they have one thing in common— the ocean. The ocean's minerals, in combination with the sun, rejuvenate the body and restore vitality, The sea is a great healer and ally. If you can, go have a swim—and breathe the ocean mist for negative ions.

    Enjoy water. Go to a spring and experience where the water comes from. Wade in a freshwater stream, river or ocean and focus your thoughts on the blessings of this element that will renew and refresh your mind.

When you go to areas where water is scarce, note how the people living there venerate water, and carry that same respect for water home with you.

Have gratitude for all the waters you come across, even Dasani.

Fire (Sunlight)

Sunlight boosts the body's supply of vitamin D. According to NCBI reports, Vitamin D deficiency is an unrecognized epidemic among both children and adults in the United States. Vitamin D deficiency not only causes rickets among children but also precipitates and exacerbates osteoporosis among adults. Vitamin D deficiency has been associated with increased risks of deadly cancers, cardiovascular disease, multiple sclerosis, rheumatoid arthritis, and type 1 Diabetes Mellitus. Those who live without adequate sunshine should supplement with vitamin D3. Regular vitamin D supplements are not received nearly as well. Vitamin D3 will promote mood and well-being during long winters and after long office days. (For more information: https://www.ncbi.nlm.nih.gov/pmc/articles/PMC3356951/)

Strangely, exposure to sunlight or daylight also helps you sleep better. Dan Pardi, researcher at the Behavioral Sciences Dept of Stanford University, says we are not getting enough bright light exposure during the day, and then in the evening we are getting too much artificial light exposure. Both of those have the consequence of causing our rhythms to get out of sync. (See dansplan.com at https://www.humanos.me/)

Pardi says the first 30-60 minutes of outdoor light exposure creates about 80% of the anchoring effect. It seems the less morning light you expose yourself to, the more difficult it will be for you to fall asleep and wake up at your set time.

According to the National Institute of Health, another benefit of sunlight exposure is that it can naturally increase the serotonin levels in your body, making you more active and alert. Getting some sun may also shake off the wintertime blues: Research suggests that light hitting your skin, not just your eyes, helps reverse seasonal affective disorder (SAD). Moreover, being outside gets us engaged in physical activity, all good. We should, however, stay out of the noon day sun and wear a good hat and shades if we must go out in the middle of the day. (https://www.ncbi.nlm.nih.gov/pmc/articles/PMC2290997/)

A serious impact of too much technology consumption and digital device use is that it is keeping us inside and also exposing our eyes to damage from blue light exposure. Blue light is harmful, because it's the highest energy wavelength of visible light. This energy is also able to penetrate all the way to the back of the eye, through the eyes' natural filters. The effects of blue light are cumulative and can lead to eye diseases like macular degeneration. Children are especially at risk as their eyes are still developing and they don't have protective pigments to help filter out some of the harmful light.

There are now apps that control the blue light on your screen and lenses that filter out blue light. The lenses have little-to-no tint and can help to minimize the direct blue light exposure that you get throughout the day. If you cannot limit your digital device use, at least cut back on it before bedtime. Accordingly to the *Harvard Health Letter* 2012, it suppresses melatonin and delays deep REM sleep significantly. (https://www.health.harvard.edu/staying-healthy/blue-light-has-a-dark-side)

In the world of plants, note how they open their stomata in the morning and late afternoon to absorb nutrients. Sun energy is circulating in the fluids of plants and we benefit from eating fresh food out of the garden. The chlorophyll in plant tissues is one of the important ways to cleanse the body.

- Spend time in the morning and late afternoon sun
- Make sun tea using your favorite herb tea.
- Limit your blue light exposure.

Earth

Hardcore Health: Live Young!

In many ways, we have to just put the fruits of the table of the earth into our bodies and we are well. The more fresh food the better. Almost everything in nature is a superfood, some are just marketed better than others. Every wild edible berry is a nutritional storehouse of perfectly assimilated vitamins, minerals and enzymes. Every green herb has its use along with every root vegetable. If you look at some of the most brilliant thinkers on health, one of the standouts is Hippocrates. His oath "Let thy food be thy medicine" could have saved us all a lot of trouble.

Animals use plants, earth, and even insects in ways that aren't just about getting energy or nutrients, but are specifically aimed at keeping themselves and their offspring healthy. In her book *How Animals Keep Themselves Well and What We Can Learn From Them*, author Cindy Engel, of the Open University, shows that most animals routinely use a variety of techniques to deal with injury, infection, parasites and biting insects. Compared with their domesticated counterparts, such as sheep that need constant de-worming treatments a year, surveys have found wild animals are remarkably healthy, muscled and lean, with few parasites.

Chimpanzees and gorillas swallow rough leaves and fibrous plants to purge their intestines of parasites. And chimps plagued by roundworm infections have been known to eat plants with anti-parasitic properties, despite their bitter flavor and lack of nutritional value. It is not uncommon to see grazing animals eating a poisonous plant intuitively to cure themselves of a disease. Ever see your dog eating grass? Every medicinal plant contains powerful alkaloids that represent some of its bitter taste but also its healing potentials. Many of the most potent medicines in nature are also the most bitter. The knowledge of how to prepare these plants was, and is still, a birthright to the people of this earth.

Many will search for a new product to satisfy their health needs when they could spend that same money on greens, vegetables and herbs. After journeying into the world of superfoods, I found one message repeated throughout—EAT YOUR GREENS! Digging deeper into green foods, you see that any culture lacking greens in their daily diet are host to many maladies of health. Greens contain more valuable nutrients than any other food group. Unfortunately, many of these nutrients are reduced when greens are overcooked and many are lost when not thoroughly chewed.

By blending green smoothies, we unlock the true power of greens. By simply blending one bunch of kale, lettuce, spinach, or chard with some bananas, seasonal fruits and water, we create a life-changing concoction that will lead us swiftly along the road to health. People are constantly trying to up their energy with caffeinated products and syrupy energy drinks, but these drinks provide a spike of energy followed by a dramatic drop-off. Green drinks, on the other hand, provide us with abundant energy often lasting through the day. Green smoothies fill the belly and this makes them excellent for dieting and cleansing. They provide us with essential amino acids that break down into proteins once in the body.

Kristi Crowe, spokeswoman for the Institute of Food Technologists, a Chicago-based science society, says spinach is one of the great green vegetables to use in smoothies. Celery, kale, beet leaves, cucumbers and parsley are other good green vegetables or plant parts to use. Those vegetables blend well with green apples and kiwi fruit, says Crowe, as do carrots and beets that add a boost of nutrients. Crowe encourages using more vegetables than fruits in smoothies as veggies have an abundant amount of antioxidants and less sugar than fruits.

By having a salad and a green smoothie every day, we take in nearly all necessary vitamins and minerals and an abundance of chlorophyll—essentially liquid-based sun energy. Without chlorophyll, no life is possible. It cleanses our organs and fights non-beneficial bacteria, fungal infections and cancer cells. Chlorophyll carries oxygen, thereby supporting the beneficial bacteria in our intestines. These friendly little guys are responsible for breaking down our food and extracting nutrients necessary for bodily function.

To experience the highest level of our health potential we must strive to take in a wide variety of green foods in their raw form and green powder supplements on a daily basis. Klamath Blue Green Algae is my favorite when I travel and don't have a kitchen handy. I mix it with organic apple juice. It is high in B vitamins, chlorophyll, and minerals, and dramatically increases my energy and focus.

The herbs and foods I've found most effective for cleansing and nourishing the body and raising energy both creatively and emotionally are:

Green Foods: Marine phytoplankton, bee pollen, blue green algae, maca, cacao, goji, turmeric, chaga mushrooms, young coconuts, greens, citrus, berries, and any fruits and vegetables with high water content.

Many of the green foods we eat contain vitamins and minerals and other key catalysts of life. And at the very base of the chlorophyll molecule is magnesium. Most green plants are also valuable sources of vitamins both C and A, as well as D, the key to sunshine, plus phosphorus and calcium. Soup with added green, leafy vegetables, beans broths, sea vegetable and whole fish soups are excellent ways of ingesting calcium.

We can get a supply of chlorophyll by adding green smoothies to our diets, cultivating and juicing wheatgrass, micro greens, taking in green powder from cereal grasses such as barley grass, wheatgrass and others, and also supplementing our diet with Klamath Blue-Green Algae, spirulina, or chlorella. You can add them to your diet with Nori rolls for vegetable and sushi rolls. Spirulina and wakame can be used in soup broths to provide powerful ocean minerals that our bodies may lack.

According to Dr. Joseph Pizzorno, co-author of the *Encyclopedia of Natural Medicine,* and co-founder of Bastyr University, seaweeds like kelp and kombu are good sources of iodine. Make sure the seaweed you buy is certified organic. Iodine is required to produce thyroid hormones, and if levels are too low people suffer hypothyroidism. The incidence of clinical and sub-clinical hypothyroidism affects 10-15% of the population especially women. Low iodine levels in fetuses and children leads to impaired mental development and research shows an increase of fibrocystic breast disease and breast cancer.

Grass-fed Beef, Free Range Chicken and Eggs, Wild Caught Salmon

As a source of B vitamins, beef is hard to beat. A 3-ounce serving has 2.51 micrograms of B-12 and 0.08 milligrams of thiamine, whereas 3 ounces of chicken has 0.25 micrograms of B-12 and 0.06 milligrams of thiamine.

Grass-fed beef comes from cattle that eat only grass and other forage foods, and not a cheaper diet of GMO grains and other byproducts. Beef that is certified grass-fed has not been raised in confinement and has never been fed antibiotics or growth hormones. These hormones and anti-bodies have no place in the human body. They can disrupt digestive flora, thereby causing inflammatory diseases. I also recommend sticking to free range chicken and eggs and wild-caught Alaskan salmon when possible.

Grass-fed beef has less fat than conventional beef, 50 percent more omega-3 fatty acids and four times more conjugated linoleic acid which reduces the risk of arteriosclerosis and improves lean body mass. Grass-fed beef is also richer in antioxidants. (Read more at: https://www.mayoclinic.org/diseases-conditions/heart-disease/expert-answers/grass-fed-beef/faq-20058059)

Studies suggest that grass-fed beef contains fewer bacteria that can cause food poisoning. Consumer Reports in 2015 tested 300 samples of beef purchased from stores across the United States and determined that beef from conventionally raised cows was three times as likely as grass-fed beef to contain bacteria resistant to multiple antibiotics. The report recommended that consumers choose grass-fed beef whenever possible.

According to USDA data, a small fillet of wild salmon has 131 fewer calories and half the fat content of the same amount of farmed salmon. And although farmed salmon may have slightly more omega-3 fatty acids, it also has 20.5 percent more saturated fat. Many consumer guides say that regardless of how it is raised, some fish is better than no fish. In other words, don't stop eating fish just because it is farm-raised or not wild-caught.

However, Mary Ellen Camire, professor of Food Science and Human Nutrition at the University of Maine's School of Food and Aquaculture, strongly advises that consumers be leery of some international farm-raised products, mostly because other countries have different standards.
(https://umaine.edu/foodandagriculture/camire2/)

Your Digestive System and Staying Young

The other missing part of a typical diet is a focus on digestive health. We have millions of microflora in the stomach and intestines, and we can only absorb vitamins and minerals into our bloodstreams with their help. These are the true warriors of health and they need all the support we can give them. The reason we're supposed to take probiotic supplements is to replace the probiotics that people used to get in a wide range of unprocessed fermented foods such as homemade yogurt, yogurt with active cultures, sauerkraut, buttermilk, pickled foods, kimchi, real soy sauce, raw vinegar, tempeh, etc

Processing and cooking destroy enzymes in food. Any sustained heat of approximately 1180 - 1290 F destroys virtually all enzymes. Read more from Jon Barron, author of *The Miracle Doctors,* 2002. (http://www.alternativehealth.co.nz/cancer/enzmes.htm)

This means that, for most of us, the food entering our stomach is severely enzyme-deficient and sits there like a heavy lump, with very little pre-digestion taking place. This forces the body to produce large amounts of stomach acid in an attempt to overcompensate. Eventually, your body's capacity to produce stomach acid begins to fade. As a result, food is insufficiently processed. This results in partial digestion of food, leading to gas, bloating, belching, food allergies, diarrhea/constipation, autoimmune disorders, skin diseases, rheumatoid arthritis, and a host of intestinal disorders such as Crohn's and IBS.

Digestive enzyme supplements give the body a chance to rest and recover its ability to produce sufficient stomach acid. Also recommended is one teaspoon of apple cider vinegar with water and a little honey taken with every meal.

Drinking aloe vera juice every day may help soothe irritated tissue and help balance out digestive juices in the stomach. (See more at https://www.ncbi.nlm.nih.gov/books/NBK92765/)

Fermented foods are found in every indigenous culture. A good probiotic supplement and fermented foods encourage a wide army of beneficial bacteria in the intestines. (Read more at: https://www.ncbi.nlm.nih.gov/pmc/articles/PMC4923703/)

Digestive enzymes play a key role in taking digestive burdens off the body. Enzymes that break down heavy metals can work towards accelerating cellular rejuvenation. This alone can be beneficial in slowing some of the effects of aging. A great digestive enzyme called aspergillus oryzae can be found in vegetarian enzyme supplements.

A major problem we face is in the way we farm. All of the topsoil in our country has been stripped for decades. The soil-borne bacteria is often completely stripped and devoid in the farms of today. These bacteria were part of the human diet for thousands of years before technological advancements and industry. Once we made the mechanical plow, our stomachs were never to be the same. Scientists today are finding that organisms once inhabited topsoil and were absorbed in trace amounts with the foods that made it into people's diets. They provide a backbone for digestive flora and are becoming rarer and rarer in modern-day agriculture. To get these flora into the body, it is important to consume a probiotic that has a wide range of beneficial bacteria.

Dr. B.J. Hardick, founder of the Centre for Maximized Living in London, Ontario, says most people are unfortunately unaware of several other incredible, and typically better, sources of healthy gut bacteria. (See: http://www.drhardick.com/probiotics-healthy-digestion)

Supplementing the diet with fermented foods like kimchi, sauerkraut, yogurt, Kefir, green peas (raw), miso, kombucha, Umeboshi plums, pickles, cheese (soft fermented like Parmesan, Gouda, Swiss), and tempeh is an excellent way to build up these bacteria. Lack of digestive enzyme production will lead to common digestive complaints, says enzyme expert Tom Bohager. T. Bohager, author of *Enzymes: What the Experts Know*.

Eating raw foods can help, but such enzyme amounts usually are only sufficient to digest the foods in which they are found. Most of us don't even get these quantities, thanks to cooking and processing. Enzyme supplements that provide the most variety are usually the best. We recommend choosing an enzyme formula with not only a high potency, but also with a high variety of enzymes. Different enzymes perform different and important functions. It is best to find a formula with multiple strains of the same enzyme in order to get the most out of that particular enzyme. When digestive problems are more chronic, a more comprehensive blend may be in order. In this case, you would want an enzyme blend that includes additional proteases, lactase, cellulase, hemicellulase and possibly alpha-galactosidase.

Hardcore Health: Live Young!

Today many raw foods that are not organic are energetically altered or irradiated for longer shelf life, killing the enzymes. Also, our bodies have to break down 100% of cooked and processed food.

Dr Howell, enzyme research pioneer, recommends chewing food longer as saliva has an enzyme called amylase. He also recommends taking enzyme supplements between meals on an empty stomach. This will go directly to the bloodstream and clean up the blood, including fat and protein deposits left in your artery walls and sludge in your colon and intestines. Dr Howell says if you take three enzyme capsules every day on an empty stomach, the additional benefits are so numerous they would be a shame to miss. They free up the metabolic enzymes and immune system from cleaning up undigested particles so they can go back to repairing and protecting your body. (https://www.westonaprice.org/health-topics/nutrition-greats/edward-howell-md/)

CHAPTER 7—HOW TO GROW YOUR OWN

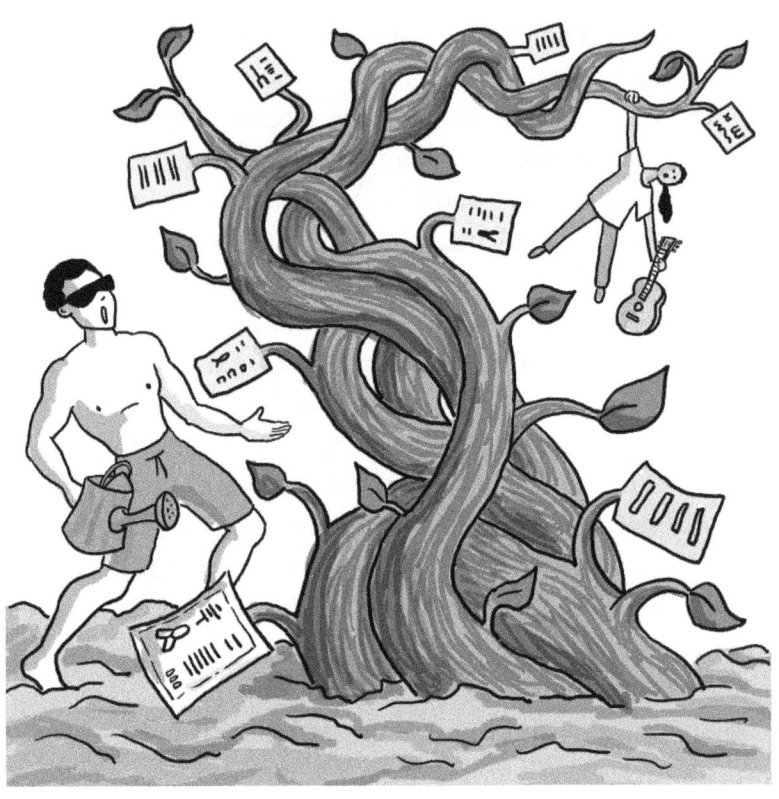

REASONS TO GROW YOUR OWN
One of the most rewarding things I've ever done is grow my own vegetables. By growing your own, you can ensure you and your family are eating nutritious and pesticide-free vegetables.

Hardcore Health: Live Young!

Several studies suggest that our food today is less nutritious than it was in the past because soil is depleted of minerals. Some high-yielding plants are also less nutritious than historical varieties. Other issues include extensive use of chemical fertilizers and the prevalence of GMO foods. A 2004 study evaluated Department of Agriculture data for 43 garden crops from 1950 to 1999. The researchers found statistically reliable declines for six nutrients: protein, calcium, potassium, iron and vitamin C. (http://hortsci.ashspublications.org/content/44/1/15.full)

One way to be sure you're getting good vegetables growing in good soil is to grow your own. You don't need a farm or a big backyard necessarily to do this. You can start off small with mega-nutritious sprouts.

Here's how to do it and do it well, no matter if you live in a condo or on a farm.

SPROUTING

Bean sprouts, micro greens, sunflower greens, buckwheat greens, broccoli sprouts, radish sprouts, wheatgrass and many great kitchen herbs can be grown indoors, in plastic trays on sunny window sills. This diversity of herbs, greens, grasses, and sprouts is a great addition to the fresh living foods in your daily diet.

Sprouts are sold at grocery stores and markets. So buy locally at farmers' markets or, for ultimate freshness, grow or sprout your own. You can keep a continuous supply available at home by growing them yourself. This same method can be used to grow broccoli, alfalfa, clover, radish, sunflower, and many other small seeded sprouts.

Supplies

Here's what you need:

1. Organic seeds marked for sprouting. This is important. Don't buy ordinary, chemically sprayed seeds.

2. Potting soil.

3. Shallow containers, like trays for planting. The containers needed for planting the broccoli seeds can be recycled items like berry containers, or you can use baking pans, lined cardboard boxes or anything that will hold a layer of soil and keep it moist.

4. Plastic wrap.

How to Sprout Seeds

1. Soak the seeds overnight in room temperature water.

2. Place a layer of soil in the container and add a bit of water to moisten.

3. Scatter a thin layer of seeds on top of the soil. You don't need to worry about spacing the

seeds out, since they won't be growing into full plants.

    4. Cover the seeds with a thin layer of potting soil.

    5. Place a layer of plastic wrap over the top of the container, and poke a few holes in the plastic to allow for gentle air circulation.

    6. Store in a warm, dry place away from direct sunlight. Place in indirect sunlight and remove plastic cover when sprouts almost touch it.

    Three to five days after sprouting, your sprouts should be ready to eat. Sprout seeds every few days in a new container to keep up a continuous supply.

    Sunflower sprouts, grown in the same way, grow about 4 inches high and are the most delicious sprout by far.

    The Sprouting Book by Ann Wigmore covers all the things you need to know to grow a wide variety of sprouts. You'll be off to a good start once you start growing your thriving sprouts. According to Johns Hopkins University, 3-day-old broccoli sprouts, for example, contain as much as 50 times the amount of some of the health-boosting phytonutrients of the mature broccoli head. Both forms of broccoli provide Vitamin A and Vitamin C. Broccoli sprouts are a better source of Vitamin K, with nearly 38 micrograms per half-cup serving. Sulphoraphane, a compound with purported anticancer and anti-diabetic properties, is present in high concentrations in 3- to 4-day-old broccoli sprouts. (See further interesting information on sprouts on website: https://sproutpeople.org/sprouts/nutrition/science/)

BALCONY AND PATIO HERB GARDENS

Balconies and patios are excellent spots to grow a supply of fresh herbs. Herbs like basil, oregano, parsley, mint, rosemary, and thyme can be tossed into salads, used in sauces, and added to flavor meats and fish. Chives are also easy to grow in pots, and great in cooking and salads. Spearmint, peppermint, mint, and chamomile make popular teas. Many flowers, such as pansies, nasturtiums and marigolds, are beautiful and edible. Herbs are grown for cooking, healing, fragrance, and garden display.

Fragrant herbs like mint and germander can be used to clear the air and freshen breath. Mint is a stimulant that revives tired feet when used in a foot spa. Two parts of baking soda mixed with one part dried lavender flowers, sprinkled and then vacuumed, deodorizes a carpet.

Herbs are one of the easiest plants to grow. A starter plant of Genovese Basil in a well-drained pot is a good beginning. Repot three basil plants in a 10 gallon pot and you will have basil all summer.

Some herbs are annual and some are perennial plants. Annual herbs are grown for one season, harvested when flower buds develop, and then discarded at the end of the season. Perennial herbs grow year after year and can be brought indoors during a chilly winter if needed.

Sunlight is essential when growing herbs. Most of our culinary herbs come from the Mediterranean and other sunny regions, so they will need a spot with sunlight at least eight hours a day. Growing herbs indoors requires a very sunny south-facing windowsill, but that still won't be as good as growing the plant outdoors. However, I studied growing herbs at the California School of Herbal Studies in a fairly cool and shady forest area of Northern California and the place was fragrant with herbs.

Herbs can be grown in any type of container with drainage holes. Large pots with large drainage holes are best as herbs can't stand having their roots sitting in too wet soil. Use loose, well-drained potting mix. A mixture of herbs and flowers can be planted in one container. It's better to combine two or more plants in a large pot than to use several little pots.

Water the soil in the pot until it starts to drip from the drainage holes. Do not over-fertilize herbs. Pinch the tips of the plants during the growing season to keep them bushy and compact. Remove any dead or diseased leaves. Because the potting mix in a pot dries out quickly, you will need to water frequently. Check by sticking your finger into the soil. If it feels dry an inch beneath the surface, it's time to water. Most delicate herbs require moderate and regular watering. This is particularly true during hot summer months. If you have good drainage at the bottom of your pot with a drainage hole and possibly rocks beneath the soil, it will be difficult to water herbs too much.

Unless the soil mix comes with slow release fertilizer, you will need to replenish the soil with fertilizer. Use a regular houseplant fertilizer at one-half the strength recommended on the label every three weeks or so. Or add a slow-release or organic fertilizer when you plant.

You can buy herb seeds or herb plants. Small herb plants are available in garden centers and these are easiest to grow. Gently spread the roots when you're planting, and cover the roots with potting mix, firming around the roots. Water immediately.

Plant seeds based on number of plants per container and planting depth depending on seed size. Water immediately after planting the seeds.

Let's return to your basil growing happily in a pot on your patio. To get your best crop, harvest and cut back the plant before it grows flowers. Harvest by removing top leaves and stems with a sharp knife. Cut the herb just above a set of growing leaves. Leave the big leaves at the bottom alone and take from the tender top new leaves of the plant. When harvesting basil and annual leafy herbs, leave four to six inches of shoots on the plant for better re-growth. Trim your basil regularly or it will continue to grow straight up and become too tall and top-heavy. Making your first trim approximately four inches above the soil produces a nice sturdy plant. As it continues to grow, continue to prune it approximately every four inches for a bushy, strong plant. After growing for some time you can cut back to three inches of the original cut which should give you plenty of basil for pesto sauce.

BACKYARD GARDENS
Garden Beds

One of the best ways to make a small space productive is by using raised garden beds. Usually two 6ft boards and two 10ft boards are nailed together creating a long rectangular bed. The boards can be approximately a foot high depending on width of wood. It is important to use non-pressure-treated wood as pressure-treated has toxic chemicals added to preserve the wood. Fill these beds with quality organic topsoil or compost, and then plant. Backyard gardens, made with raised beds, with double-dug or sheet mulch methods are very productive and well designed. The raised bed double-dug method is discussed in an incredibly useful book called *How to Grow More Vegetables* by John Jeavons.

The sheet mulch method is used often in permaculture and widely discussed online. Sheet mulch makes use of yard waste (leaves, pesticide-free grass clippings, and mulch under) and recycled materials like cardboard, newspaper and other items usually sent to the dump. By being resourceful, we can find these items in neighbors' yards and our own; most of the time, people are happy to help you out if you ask. Sheet mulch gardens are great because they require very little maintenance and get better with age. The ground weeds are cut and are suppressed by the cardboard and manure in the bottom of the bed. The beds remain relatively free of weeds as long as weed seeds aren't in the material used to make the beds. The plants can be planted in little pockets of potting soil you make amidst the mulch and green materials.

There are many incredible gardening methods like sheet mulch discussed at www.permacultureglobal.org. The art of permaculture, presented by Bill Mollison in his series of books, is an effective way to save our planet by mimicking nature in designs. It covers methods of gardening, building, and water management that will be very useful in the future of our troubled climate.

Good Soil Feeds You and Your Plants

In the raised bed method, quality planting soil can be bought in bags or delivered to your door. Boxes filled with quality organic soil and compost can be put into immediate use, as long as you enrich it with plenty of compost and finish with a thick layer of mulch (leaves, grass clipping, woodchips) from 2 - 6 inches deep. This mulch protects soil life, conserves water, and prevents weeds growing. This process is simple and rewarding, and saves newbies the trouble of amending and working the existing backyard soil that could be poor, polluted, or very hard and labor intensive to dig. These growing beds can be put directly on lawns or even weeds, if a thick underneath layer of soaking wet cardboard is used to kill off grass or weeds.

It's extremely important to have good soil to nourish and nurture your plants so they in turn will nourish and nurture you. With good soil and nutrition, plants grow healthy and become naturally resistant to disease and insect pests. Strong plants form much higher levels of alkaloids and essential oils making them unappealing to insects and bugs. Insects are looking for vulnerable, weak plants that are closer to decaying.

It is well worth starting a compost pile or a worm bin to make use of valuable food scraps and yard waste. A well composted garden is teeming with microbes and organic matter, the building blocks of healthy soil. This is when food becomes medicine—one of the best reasons to grow your own.

Manure, compost, and mulch are used to quickly restore life to the soil. Adding compost to soil balances the pH, dramatically increases pest resistance and enhances nutrition. It makes everything grow better, as does a generous layer of mulch, which in time becomes compost. Adding compost or compost tea or manure to the garden is the best way to simply make great plants grow. You can add organic matter to your soil with compost, shredded leaves, animal manures, or cover crops. Organic matter provides a continuous source of nitrogen and other nutrients that plants need to grow.

    Rock Dust, like azomite, gypsum dolomite, crushed basalt and calcium carbonate, is another beneficial addition to soil, providing abundant minerals for you via your plants. By adding additional micronutrients like boron, zinc, iron, and silica in recommended quantities, we can in turn assimilate them into our bodies via our vegetables and fruits.

    This can only be achieved through a detailed soil analysis, but is truly the cutting edge of nutrition. Look at the work of Jana Bogs in her book *Beyond Organic* for more information on soil tests and amending soil. I feel, however, that a person new to gardening should focus on composting, adding rock dust, and hold off on detailed soil analysis until they are trying to perfect their process

Trellising

    If you are growing in a small space, you want to grow as many crops as possible on vertical supports. Indian teepees, built with three long sticks of bamboo or similar tied at the top, will support climbing varieties of peas and pole beans. Other vegetables that are commonly trellised include vining crops such as cucumbers and tomatoes. The fence surrounding your back garden may well do double-duty as a trellis.

    I think it is great to have a big vision for the garden, of getting it fertile and productive. It is, however, very important to start small. Choose just a few of your favorite veggies for a start. There are so many things to know, but don't be discouraged easily; you'll never learn your environment's unique challenges until you start trying.

What to Grow and When to Grow It

    For your first try, you may want to buy seedlings, as some veggies are notoriously difficult to grow from seed. However, beans, corn, summer and winter squash, carrots, beets, spring mixes of greens, Asian greens, and many more grow well from directly sowed seeds. As a good rule of thumb, if the seed has a very close spacing listed for planting, sow the seeds direct and thin out the extras as directed. If the seed has a wide spacing of 6 inches or more, sow them in trays and plant them out when they have developed, or buy them from a garden center ready to transplant. It is labor intensive to transplant, but well worth the head start.

If you grow winter squash, beans, and corn, you can train the beans to grow up the corn and the squash will keep the weeds from coming up too much. This method is called "The Three Sisters." It is an age-old Native American technique for maximizing production in a small space. There are many different combinations of plants you can plant in close proximity that will actually support each other. These are called "plant guilds" or companion plantings. They involve using flowers and herbs that may repel insects mixed with productive crops and groundcovers. They can be very beautiful.

One could grow mint, basil, chard and cucumbers in the same area, and plant marigolds to repel bugs away from the cucumbers. Basil repels aphids, flies, mosquitoes, mites and hornworms that attack tomatoes. Lavender repels slugs. Many pests find the smell of marigolds repulsive and they also produce a chemical that is toxic to parasitic worms, so these are an excellent addition to your garden.

It's a good idea to plant the garden bit by bit by planting something new almost every week of the season. This makes planting less of a chore and works well for harvesting a constant supply of fresh food. When your crop is one month from maturity, start new transplants to replace what has been harvested. In this way you will keep a rotation of fresh veggies. Fill in gaps with quick, easy-to-grow-from-seed crops like radish, turnips, salad mixes, and Asian greens. Living mulches, like white clover and buckwheat, are also great ways to fill in gaps and suppress weeds.

Spring—Cool Season Crops:
Lettuce (harvest as you trim for constant source of fresh greens,) sugar peas, beans, radish, Swiss chard, summer squash, zucchini, rhubarb, chives, and kale.

Summer—Warm Season Crops:
Corn, eggplant, peppers, tomatoes and cherry tomatoes, basil, and strawberries.

Most of these plants are delicious enough to pop right into your mouth, so you're nourishing your body as you exercise it in your garden.

PART 3—WHOLESOME AND DELICIOUS RECIPES FROM KATIE'S TROPICAL KITCHEN

Katie Amato is the author of recipes on *Katie's Tropical Kitchen,* katiestropicalkitchen.com. She has a B.S. in Cognitive Psychology and Masters in Public Health (M.P.H.), with a focus on social and behavioral health behavior change, and a particular interest in growing, cooking and teaching others about delicious, nutritious, and fresh food. She is the co-author of several peer-reviewed journal publications and book chapters relating to physical activity, inactivity, and nutrition.

Her recipes found in this collection focus on fresh, whole ingredients. Although, not emphasized in individual recipes, the use of organic, unprocessed, non-GMO, and local (when possible) ingredients are highly encouraged. Most of these recipes use whole foods, which do not even require a nutrition label because it is the most pure form of the food. Cooking in this manner ensures you are in control of what goes into your body, that your contact with pesticides and herbicides is reduced, and that the maximum nutrition available in these foods goes straight into your dish.

It is important to use healthy and quality products, and cooking methods. It is just as important to use food that has been stored properly and cookware that is non-toxic. Equally important are cleaning products like dish soap and hand soap.

BEVERAGES: DRINK YOUR VITAMINS.
The Green Green Smoothie

Equipment: High horsepower blender.

First, add 1-2 inches of water just above the blades in the blender jar.

Then pick 1-2 of the following leafy greens: 1-2 cups salad greens, 1 cup spinach, 1 small head lettuce, 4-6 leaves of kale

Then add in some other green vegetables: ½ zucchini, 1 stalk celery, 1/2 cucumber. Also, add some creamy fruits.

Pick one or more of these types of creamy fruits to make your smoothie smooth: 1-4 small bananas (frozen works well but fresh is ok too), 1/2 avocado, eggfruit, sapote (mamey sapote, chicos).

Additionally, you can add other fruits for extra taste and sweetness:1 apple, 1/2 cup ripe jackfruit, 1/2 cup mango, 1-2 passion fruit.

Then, think about other superfood additions to boost your smoothie with extra nutrition. Add a serving or two of the following: microalgae, chlorella, spirulina, flaxseed, hemp seed, soaked chia seeds, maca powder, goji berries, bee pollen, shredded coconut.

I recommend getting used to having smoothies that are less sweet, but if the smoothie isn't sweet enough for you add a little honey, maple syrup or stevia.

To get the most out of your green smoothie it is best to use a blender with a high horsepower at maximum speed. It ionizes all the nutrients so that you body absorbs them instantly. We use a 3 horsepower Blendtec blender.

With water, fill the first 1-2 inches in the blender jar, add the greens first, then pile on other veggies and fruits. To make more room in the blender, "pulse" it until the greens are chopped. Add the rest of your selection of ingredients and a few ice cubes to cool it down a little. Blend on high for two 30-second intervals.

Choco-Banana Flax Smoothie

Fiber is crucial for our diets. Flax seed not only has a high fiber content, but it also has high omega-3 fatty acid content, lignans which have antioxidant properties, and their mucilage (gummy when ground and mixed with liquid) content helps them remain in the stomach longer to absorb nutrients. Raw cacao powder also has many antioxidants and natural caffeine, so you can feel good about this smoothie, for breakfast, lunch, or dinner.

Servings: 2
Ingredients:
2 medium bananas
2 tablespoons flax

2 tablespoons raw chocolate powder
6 ice cubes
1/2 cup water, almond milk, rice milk or other substitute
Optional sweetener like honey, maple syrup or stevia to taste

Steps: Blend everything together on high in intervals of 30 seconds. Add sweetener if desired, and chill if not cool enough.

Carrot Apple Beet Ginger Juice

What a name, huh? The name lists the ingredients in order of quantity that make up this luscious cleansing juice. This carrot apple beet ginger juice is so satisfying. Drinking fresh vegetable and fruit juices is a great way to deliver nutrients to your body. It is an ideal addition to your diet because these nutrients can be absorbed better and faster than if you were eating the vegetables and juices. However, juicing removes most of the beneficial fiber you would normally be consuming by eating, instead of drinking, the produce.

Many people have varying opinions on juicing. Especially, on juice cleanses. I personally have found short juice cleanses to be extremely effective. I did my first 3-day juice cleanse as a last resort to bronchial sickness. An urgent care clinician prescribed me antibiotics, which were not effective. Desperate for a solution, a friend recommended a juice fast. The idea is that it delivers nutrients to your system fast while giving you digestive system (and your whole body) a break. This break from your digestive system is helpful because your body is able to route your resources towards curing your illness. After 3 short days, my sickness was gone.

Since then, I've done a few more juice fasts/cleanses. At the end, I felt brilliant and my mental fogginess was gone. I felt extreme emotional and mental clarity, and had increased energy. This carrot apple ginger juice is a standby for me.

Yield: almost 4 cups, 32 ounces.

Equipment: juicer

Ingredients (organic!!):

10-15 large carrots (tops cut off)

3 small apples (cored, not peeled)

⅓ of a very large beet (size of an large orange), or ½ of a medium beet (tennis ball), 1 whole small beet (peeling it gives it a cleaner flavor)

1 inch piece of ginger (peeled)

Steps:

Wash all ingredients, peel if needed. Start with the carrots and juice until you get about 2 cups of juice. Add the apples, and then the beet until you get a nice red pinkish color. Add the ginger and juice and a few more carrots until you get the desired amount of juice. Taste and add more of the above to adjust for any other flavors.

Fresh Green Vegetable Juice with Apple

Hardcore Health: Live Young!

This fresh green juice recipe is great for the morning, refreshing, and so healthy. Although there is some fruit, it is still a fresh vegetable juice. There are several reasons why it is super healthy for you. The Vitamin C in the lemon helps you to absorb the iron from the greens. The apples make it just sweet enough. It is made with several ingredients that you are likely to have on hand: celery, cucumber, lettuce, lemon, apples. You can feel free to substitute the lettuce for more greens, etc.

Yield: Makes about 3 cups of juice

Equipment: Any standard vegetable juicer

Ingredients:

2-4 stalks of celery

1 bunch (8-12 leaves) kale (can remove stems for less bitter taste)

1 large cucumber

½ head lettuce

½ lemon, peeled and seeded

2-4 apples (the amount depends on apple's size and your sweet tongue)

1 small-medium zucchini (optional)

Steps: Feed the cucumber and zucchini pieces through the juicer, alternating with the kale and the lettuce. Add the lemon. Then add the celery last because the fibers tend to clog juicers.

Watermelon Mint Juice

The recipe is for fresh watermelon mint juice that you don't have to juice! This is such a refreshing beverage with multiple health benefits. In Chinese medicine, watermelon is a cooling food, which reduces heat signs and helps the yin and blood sugar imbalances. Watermelon helps to relieve you from summer heat. It is also used to help treat depression, inflammations of the kidney and urinary tract system, edema, and treats thirst and dehydration.

Furthermore, it helps to build body fluids and moistens intestines. Watermelon is alkalizing, which means it helps reduce acidic conditions and inflammation, making it less likely that disease will take hold in your body. When cutting up your melon, don't be afraid to get close to and include some of the rind (if it's organic). The rind contains a compound known as citrulline. Citrulline helps protect against free-radical damage and converts into arginine (an important amino acid that helps dilate your blood vessels and improve circulation). If you are using a juicer, you can juice half of the rind of an organic watermelon.

Equipment: blender

Yield: 5 cups of juice

Ingredients:

1/2 small watermelon, seeds and rind removed (2 1/2 pounds, 1000g or more)

Juice of one lime

3 sprigs or more fresh mint

6 ice cubes

1/2 cup water

Steps: Deseed watermelon, remove rind, and place in blender (should be around 4 or 5 cups). Wash and place mint leaves in blender along with ice and lime juice. Blend on high for 30 seconds, taste, and adjust to taste.

SALAD AND SIDE DISHES
Simple Salad with Creamy Macadamia Nut Dressing

This creamy macadamia nut dressing recipe is Adam's creation. It is essentially one of the only dressings we make because it is so satisfying. It also has many different applications besides salad. For example, we use it mixed with pasta as the sauce, we use it in our tacos, on top of Shepherd's Pie, to dip our carrots in, and more. The texture is silky, with a slight tang, a subtle sweetness, and a strange taste resemblance to bacon. Adam says it reminds him of the secret sauce commonly used in fast food restaurants. Yet, this recipe is vegan, gluten-free, GMO-free, and extremely delicious.

Macadamia nuts are the local choice for nuts or seeds in Hawaii. They also have a unique set of nutritional benefits. It is an excellent source of energy as it has one of the highest caloric values for the seeds/nuts (100g is 718 calories). They are high in fiber and are naturally gluten-free. Additionally, macadamia nuts are packed with minerals (calcium, iron, magnesium, manganese, selenium and zinc), antioxidants, and vitamins (especially B-complex vitamins, with smaller amounts of Vitamin A and Vitamin E). Macadamia nuts are also a rich source of monounsaturated fatty acids like oleic acid and palmitoleic acid. These are known to help lower total LDL (bad) cholesterol and increase HDL or good cholesterol.

Ingredients:

1 cup mac nuts (or other creamy nut, like cashews)

1/4 cup plus 2 tablespoons soy

1/4 of a medium red bell pepper

4-6" sprig of rosemary (stem removed)

1/2 – 1/3 cup water

1/4 cup plus 2 tablespoons olive oil

3 tablespoons mustard

2 tablespoons soy

Blend ingredients together in blender, slowly adding water until creamy consistency is achieved. Add salt if necessary.

Salad:

(choose at least 3 from the below)

Chopped mixed lettuces

Chopped tomatoes

Carrot slices (use a peeler to get thin strips and make it easier to chew)

Beet slices, same method as above

Sliced radish

Chopped cucumber

Fresh corn

Sprouts

Raisins
Chopped apples

Mashed Winter Squash

Two cups cooked and mashed winter squash
1 teaspoon cinnamon
2 teaspoons coconut oil
Salt to taste
Mix together and heat in small pan or pot.
Variations: Instead of coconut oil and cinnamon, add salt and cheese, or add cumin and red chili pepper

Tomatoes with Balsamic Olive Oil and Sea Salt (or Bruschetta)

This recipe for tomatoes with fresh basil and olive oil is like the Italian Caprese salad. But you don't have to add cheese to make it taste delicious. The most important thing is fresh tomatoes and high quality olive oil. Good salt is also a huge plus! This recipe is great to share with guests when there is an abundance of tomatoes.

Ingredients:
Vine-ripened tomatoes
Balsamic Vinegar
Olive Oil
Sea salt
Fresh basil chopped
Fresh mozzarella (optional)

Steps: Slice tomatoes and place on plate so that they are not overlapping. Drizzle with balsamic vinegar and olive oil. Spread sea salt evenly and top with fresh basil and optional mozzarella.

Variation: Chop the tomatoes fine, add balsamic and olive oil and crushed garlic, and let marinade with salt and pepper. Toast small pieces of bread and top with tomato mixture and optional cheese.

Guacamole

The quickest, most-filling portion of good fat for your diet is one of the easiest to make. Just try to avoid buying chips to accompany it. Dip carrots, celery, zucchini slices, enjoy on a sandwich or on the side of your dinner plate. Serve with beans and rice for a simple, complete and healthy meal.

Yield: 1-2 cups depending on size of your avocado.

Ingredients:
1 large buttery avocado (save the seed)
¼ medium onion diced
1 tomato (diced)
½ lime (squeezed juice, hold the seeds)
Pinch or more of sea salt
Black pepper or a little chili pepper
Cilantro or cilantro substitute such as Culantro

Steps:

Mix all ingredients well. Store with the seed (to keep it from getting brown). Eat fresh or refrigerate.

Basil Macadamia Nut Pesto

Yield: about 2 cups pesto
Equipment: Blender or food processor
Ingredients:
1/2 cup olive oil
1 cup shredded parmesan cheese
1/2 cup macadamia nuts (or pine nuts, walnuts, cashews, brazil nuts).
Salt and pepper to taste
8 cups or more loosely packed basil leaves
Steps: Blend olive oil and garlic together until garlic is well chopped. Add basil, cheese, macadamia nuts and blend. Add salt and pepper to taste. Store in air-tight jar in the fridge (you can adjust the quantities as desired).

Sautéed Greens and Garlic

I know this recipe is almost too basic to write down, but I think it deserves the spotlight for a moment because of its simplicity. It is so important to eat your greens and the ease of this recipe should be an inspiration to prepare and eat greens daily with any meal.

Yield: 4 servings
Equipment: Large pan
Ingredients:

2-3 bunches of greens, like kale, Swiss chard, spinach, mustard greens, leafy cabbage, other edible greens

1 medium onion chopped or sliced

4 cloves of garlic

Olive oil

Salt

Pepper

Steps: Wash and chop greens. Heat 1 tablespoon olive oil in large sauté pan, add onion and stir frequently until translucent. Add garlic and cook for another 2 minutes stirring frequently. Then add chopped greens and stir until they reduce, and then keep adding more. Cook for 10 minutes or so, until leaves are very tender. Season with salt and pepper, and serve alongside any main meal. Variations:

Add other vegetables: diakon (absorbs the flavors well), tomatoes (helps you absorb the iron from the leafy greens), mushrooms, etc.

Shredded Carrot and Beet Salad with Tahini Dressing

If you need a good way to include more raw beets in your diet, this is it. This is a great side salad to bring to potlucks if you want to have something healthy around. People are often amazed at how delicious the beets can taste with this protein-packed dressing.

Yield: 4-6 servings

Equipment: Food processor or other method for grating beets and carrots
(example: mandoline slicer, spiralizer, cheese grater)

Ingredients for salad:
10 medium-large carrots
2-3 beets
Lettuce or mixed baby greens

Dressing ingredients:
4-6 tablespoons tahini (depending on taste)
2 medium cloves garlic, chopped
3 tablespoons balsamic vinegar
3 tablespoons olive oil
¼ cup (or more water)
1 teaspoon honey
1-2 tablespoons lemon juice
Salt to taste
(Optional: 1/2 ounce of goat cheese)

Steps: Grate the carrots and then the beets (easiest in food processor). Prepare the dressing in blender by combining all ingredients until smooth. Place the carrots and beets in a bowl and mix in the dressing, serve on top of lettuce or mixed baby greens.

Artichokes with Garlic Olive Oil Dipping Sauce

Artichokes were always a treat in my house, fun to snack on and a reason to dip something in butter. This healthier version relies on an olive oil dipping sauce instead of the traditional melted butter or even mayo. At times I sprinkle only a little sea salt on the pieces and skip the sauce all together.

Ingredients:
Artichokes
Salt
Pepper
Garlic
Olive oil

Steps: Cut the tips off of each artichoke leaf (just the tip). Place in steamer or boil until tender (usually 30 minutes or until the leaves are easily plucked out and the meat on the leaves can be scrapped off), then remove from water and drain. For dipping sauce, combine crushed garlic, olive oil, salt and pepper. Serve while still warm with dipping sauce.

LIGHT MEALS

Herbed Vegetable Frittata

Frittatas are one of my favorite meals to make for guests. They are simple, only require a few dishes, and you can add as many ingredients as you have on hand. Additionally, they are flexible, forgiving, and filling!

I see frittatas as the perfect way to get your veggies and protein into the beginning of your day. However, this is not just another breakfast dish. Of course it is great at brunch too. Yet, sometimes I also love making this for dinner (if I didn't already have eggs for breakfast). It is quick and easy and warming. Another plus is that frittatas are great eaten cold, and leftovers are the perfect snack or to-go lunch for the next day. If you want to make your frittatas a little more filling, try adding slices of boiled potato. This is most similar to the Spanish tortilla.

Adding fresh herbs to this recipe is a really good way to get some of those beneficial micronutrients from the garden. Add fresh basil, oregano, parsley, or thyme. Experiment with dill and other fresh herb favorites.

Yield: 4-6 servings

Equipment: Frying pan that is oven safe (or a frying pan and a pie plate)

Ingredients:

10-12 eggs, beaten

½ medium onion or 1 small onion chopped

2 cups chopped kale or other greens (spinach, chard, kai choy, bok choy)

Chopped fresh and ripe tomatoes (½ cup or less)

½ cup goat cheese, or shredded mozzarella, cheddar, manchego

⅓ cup chopped fresh herbs (oregano, Cuban/Mexican oregano, stick oregano, all basil, parsley, rosemary, thyme, etc.)

Optional boiled potato sliced into half-moons

1 teaspoon salt

Pepper to taste (about 30 fresh ground turns)

Steps: Preheat the oven to 350° F. First, sauté the onion (3-5 minutes) until translucent. Then, sauté the greens until wilted (3 minutes or less). Add chopped herb and sauté a few minutes longer. In a separate, medium-sized bowl, beat eggs and salt and pepper. Be careful not to under or over salt. You can start light at first and test a small bit of the egg by cooking a few drops.

Once the vegetables are cooked, add to the egg bowl and then fold in. If you are using a totally stainless steel pan with no plastic (i.e. it is 100% oven safe) then you can quickly clean it and re-oil the pan generously with olive oil or refined coconut oil. Now, you can either add the cheese to mixture or just put cheese on top in the last 5 minutes of baking. Finally, add the egg and vegetable mixture to pan. Bake immediately, about 20-25 minutes until it is clearly cooked on top, slightly brown on top, and bubbling.

Serve warm or cool.

Greens and Fruit Breakfast Bowl

Who said you can't eat salad for breakfast? Ok, it is untraditional BUT absolutely great for you, very alkaline, which not only keeps you energized and swift, but helps prevent disease from taking hold in your body. Sounds better than the way you feel after pancakes right? What really brightens up the bowl is the addition of fresh fruit and seeds.

Hardcore Health: Live Young!

If you need more carbs, eat with a healthy slice of whole-grain or gluten-free bread, add cooked quinoa or combination of cooked quinoa and millet. If you need more protein, add cheese. This recipe is another flexible, idea-creator, and game changer to start a morning with living, fresh foods. The more in-season and local, the better. If you aren't using organic, make sure to peel veggies and fruits.

Ingredients:

Start with a green base:
Baby spinach
Butter lettuce
Mānoa lettuce
Red leaf
Or mixed spring mix
Add some arugula and mizuna for a little bitter spice
Choose 2-3 fruits:
Strawberries
Grapes
Pineapple
Papaya
Apple
Orange/mandarins/clementines
Choose 2-3 veggies
Cucumber
Tomatoes
Carrots
Raw or roasted beets

Jicama

Just before serving, top with some proteins and/or fats

Sunflower seeds

Chia seed

Walnuts

Almonds

Avocado

Goat cheese

Shaved parmesan

Manchego cheese

If you need more carbs and calories:

Cooked quinoa

Whole-grain bread

Gluten-free bread

Top with a dressing:

Olive oil and vinegar

Raspberry dressing

Home-made fruit dressing (pureed fruit—like strawberries, mango, etc—vinegar, oil, and salt and pepper).

Layered Ratatouille in a Crock Pot

Ratatouille is a traditional vegetarian dish that often resembles a thick stew and is made with summer vegetables such as eggplant, tomatoes, summer squash, and onions. Bell peppers would also be a good addition. It was originally a French Provencal stewed vegetable dish from Nice. Other known names include ratatouille niçoise. The word ratatouille derives expressive forms of the French verb touiller, which means "to stir up".

This dish was also popularized by Pixar. This recipe follows the deconstructed style of ratatouille perfectly pictured in the Pixar movie. Instead of a mixed stew with chopped veggies, it is layered. I also utilize the crock pot or slow cooker to achieve the perfect level of tenderness without sacrificing the perfect, layered plating.

I suggest using the freshest local and organic ingredients available in your area. In this recipe, I use Japanese eggplants, zucchini, and tomatoes grown locally, and onions that are from a neighboring island. I also use whatever herbs are growing in my garden. To finish, add a little cheese like manchego, goat cheese, or parmesan. This layered ratatouille in a crock pot is a beautiful vegetarian dish and you can throw it together in 20 minutes or less.

Yield: 2-4 servings

Equipment: Crock pot

Ingredients:

2 medium zucchini, sliced thin
2 medium long eggplants, sliced thin
3-4 medium tomatoes, sliced thin
1 onion, sliced thin
4-6 cloves garlic
Salt, about ½ teaspoon
Pepper, about ½ teaspoon

Cheese for topping (⅓ cup shredded per person)

Herbs used in Italian cooking (about 1/3 cup chopped fresh or 1-2 tablespoons dried) oregano, basil, rosemary, thyme.

Steps: Prepare ingredients by chopping veggies and herbs (I use my food processor to slice all items, it takes so much less time than hand chopping, you could also use a mandoline). Layer zucchini, eggplant, onion, and tomato in a stack in your hand, and place in a slow-cooker (see picture). However ,there is no need to layer if you don't want to spend the time). Place the chopped herbs on top. At this point, grind in a blender (or you can chop) all the leftover vegetables, garlic and herbs, salt and pepper, and then pour on top. Season with salt and pepper. Put on low setting in slow cooker for 6-8 hours, on high for 4 hours, or a combination of the two heats. The dish is finished cooking when the vegetables are tender and aromatic. Serve topped with cheese (try manchego, sheep's milk cheese from Spain or goat cheese), and alongside pasta, bread, or as a side dish.

Cauliflower Cheddar Soup

I developed this healthy cauliflower cheddar soup recipe while visiting the east coast. This recipe comes out savory and super creamy. I don't drink milk or use cream so, unlike many recipes for this type of soup, I didn't add any extra dairy beyond the cheese. This soup is great for cheesy soup lovers who cannot tolerate the lactose in many types of cheese but can tolerate cheddar. It is also gluten-free and can be prepared vegetarian.

Yield: 4-6 servings

Equipment: Regular blender or immersion blender

Ingredients:

2 tablespoons olive oil

1 small onion, roughly chopped

2 cloves garlic roughly chopped

1 head cauliflower, cut into large florets

2-3 potatoes peeled and roughly chopped

1 quart chicken or veggie broth

1 1/2 cups shredded cheddar

Salt and pepper to taste

Steps: Sauté cauliflower, onion, potatoes, and garlic in olive oil, stirring frequently to avoid sticking. Add a little more oil as necessary to prevent sticking. Once the onions are soft, add broth (should just cover the veggies) and bring to a boil until potatoes are tender (15-30 minutes depending on how small they are chopped). Let the soup cool until it is safe to put in the blender, and then blend on high until creamy and uniform. Return to pot (rinse it out first) and heat on low. Add cheddar and stir until combined. Test it and add more salt and pepper.

Split Pea Soup

Slow cooker vegan split pea soup is comforting to eat and simple to make. It only requires a few ingredients that you are likely to have on hand. If you prefer, you don't need to make this in a slow cooker. You can cook this on the stove in 1-1.5 hours as well. You just need to be sure you keep a watch on it so that the water doesn't evaporate too quickly and burn the peas.

Yield: 4-6 servings, about 12 oz each

Equipment: Large soup pot or crock pot/slow cooker

Ingredients:

2 cups of green split peas

2 medium carrots (diced)

1 large onion (diced)

2 stalks of celery (diced)

1-2 medium potatoes (sliced into half moons)

Salt and pepper to taste

Steps: Combine ingredients into large pot or crock pot. Add water, 2 inches above veggies.

Cook for about 1-2 hours on stove top at medium heat, or 6-8 hours on high in crock pot until the peas are mushy and start to lose their shape. Be careful on the stove top to check the soup to make sure there is still enough water, and stir from time to time to prevent peas from sticking to the bottom and burning. Season with salt and pepper and serve hot.

Winter Squash Soup

Hardcore Health: Live Young!

For a while, I was convinced this soup would make people fall in love with me. In reality, I just make this soup for all the people I really truly love. This dairy-free recipe for winter squash bisque is warming, smooth, and even yummy cold. Additionally, it is quite filling, especially when served with fresh bread and/or cheese. Oh! And it is also gluten-free, vegan, and fat-free.

Depending on the variety, winter squash can have very high levels of Vitamin A (up to 350% RDV) and Vitamin C (up to 50% RDV). Look for squashes that are deeper colors of yellow, orange, and red, for example Butternut and Hubbard. These are a little higher in nutritional value than spaghetti or acorn squash. They are also loaded with fiber, and have some protein, Vitamin B6, Folate, Magnesium, Thiamin, Potassium and Manganese.

Yield: approximately 4-6 servings (about 10 oz each)

Equipment: Blender (immersion blender is the easiest) and large soup pot

Ingredients:

1 winter squash, butternut, or other medium sweet squash (medium, about 5 pounds, butternut or other creamy yellow-orange squash taste the best).

1 medium onion
1 large carrot
1 stalk of celery
1 large or 2 small potatoes

Enough water to cover ingredients (or veggie/chicken broth if you have)

Salt and pepper to taste

Steps: Cut squash open and save the seeds for planting or eating. Roast squash in the oven at 350-400° F until soft enough to scoop away the flesh from the skin easily (I put mine cut side up in a casserole dish with a little water so the steam helps it cook quicker). While squash is cooking, roughly chop the remaining ingredients. For a richer flavor, you can sauté the veggies in olive oil in a large pot for 5 minutes before you add broth or water. Then, add the water or broth until about an inch above the veggies and bring to a boil, then reduce heat to medium.

When the squash is tender, let it cool for a few minutes (so you don't burn yourself), peel it and add the chunks to the soup. Cook another 10 or so minutes to let the flavors blend. Remove from heat and let sit until it stops bubbling and the soup is cool enough to blend (you don't want a glass blender to crack under the heat, a plastic blender to melt plastic into your soup, or the immersion blender to spit up hot soup at your face and body). At this point, blend your soup until a uniform purée is achieved. Put back on the stove to warm, season with salt and pepper. Serve hot (with shredded hard cheese for some extra protein) and bread for dipping.

Tempeh with Rice and Steamed Greens

Hardcore Health: Live Young!

For a long time I thought tempeh was another health food trend, a way to sell surplus soy to the health hipsters. Furthermore, years ago I discovered that soy gave me abdominal pain, etc. It took about a year of my man insisting that it was unfermented GMO soy causing the problem. He finally convinced me that fermented organic soy, like tempeh, is healthful and delicious.

Tempeh is fermented with spores of a fungus Rhizopus oligosporus, a type of a healthy white mold that is usually high in Vitamin B and several amino acids. The Rhizopus oligosporus reduces gas and inflammation caused by soy. Tempeh has a medium-mild nutty flavor that soaks up the seasonings of the sauces it is cooked with.

This ginger tempeh recipe is quick and delicious, and it is easily prepared and served with rice and a vegetable. Try sides of steamed bok choy, sautéed kale, lettuce wraps, or a cucumber salad.

Servings: 2

Special equipment: non-stick frying pan, blender

Ingredients:
1 tablespoon sesame oil
1+ tablespoon olive oil
2 garlic cloves, roughly chopped
1 inch piece of ginger, peeled and roughly chopped
¼ of medium onion, chopped roughly
1-2 tablespoon soy sauce

1-2 teaspoons honey
¼ cup or less filtered water
1 package 8 oz organic tempeh

Steps: Blend together: garlic, ginger, onion, 1 tablespoon sesame oil, 1 tablespoon olive oil, and enough water (about ¼ cup) to easily blend the ingredients (if you want, you can use about half of this to marinate the tempeh before cooking). Slice tempeh into thin pieces about ¼ inch thick. Heat a little olive oil (teaspoon or less) in a non-stick frying pan, add tempeh in a single layer in the pan with enough room to turn them (do two batches if you have a small pan). Add sauce from the blender and turn heat to medium or medium-high and lightly "fry" each side for 3-5 minutes.

When they are starting to brown, add a "sprinkle" or tablespoon of soy sauce to the pan and a teaspoon of honey and stir until evenly distributed. Cook another 1-2 minutes until they start to brown (the soy sauce and honey will caramelize and burn if left too long). Serve with furikake rice, lettuce wraps, or bok choy.

MAIN MEALS
Baked Meatballs with Fresh Herbs

On top of spaghetti, all covered with cheese, I lost my poor meatball, when somebody sneezed. I love this little rhyme; it makes me smile every time I make meatballs. The below baked meatballs recipe was created when I went on a brief paleo diet. It features coconut flour or almond flour instead of wheat flour to thicken the meatballs.

Another special part of this recipe is that the meatballs are baked. I started baking my meatballs instead of pan-frying because it requires much less attention than constantly turning them in a pan. This means you will have plenty of time to prep a nice big salad to accompany your meal.

Also, key to this recipe is the use of a lot of herbs. I think using fresh is the best way to go. I highly recommend growing a few of your own herbs for the amazing difference in flavor and nutrients that so many recipes benefit from. If you don't have fresh herbs, you can use dried herbs, just scale back to 1-2 teaspoons total depending on the herbs you use and their strength. I also recommend using grass fed beef. Look for 100% grass-fed beef that has no unnecessary added antibiotics and hormones.

You can try serving these meatballs with my chunky basil and garlic tomato sauce and manchego cheese. My favorite accompaniment is spaghetti squash. Spaghetti squash with paleo meatballs and homemade sauce is the perfect dinner to treat your family and friends to. It is gluten-free and includes so many beautiful veggies, nutrients and proteins.

Yield: About 15 meatballs

Ingredients:

1 pound grass-fed beef (or bison!)

1/2 teaspoon sea salt or a little more to taste

Fresh pepper to taste
1/4 cup onion, diced or minced
1 small garlic clove, chopped, minced, or pressed to preference
1-2 large handfuls of fresh herbs, chopped (basil, rosemary, parsley, oregano, etc.)
1 egg beaten
1/2 cup organic white flour (one can substitute other gluten-free flours: try a flour blend or combine your own gluten-free flours, being careful that none of them dominate the flavor too much)

Steps: Preheat oven to 400° F. In a medium bowl, beat egg, add onion, garlic, salt, pepper and herbs. Then, add ground beef and mix well. Next, add flour and mix well (a few heaping tablespoons at a time so that you can mix it evenly). Form into 1 to 1 and ½ inch balls and place on ungreased cookie sheets or in shallow pans, and place in oven.

Turn every 10 minutes for 25-40 minutes until cooked to your preference (eg. medium-well).

Chunky Basil and Garlic Tomato Sauce
Yield: 8 generous servings of sauce
Ingredients:
4-5 cans organic diced tomatoes (14.5 oz)
1/2 cup red wine (optional)
8-12+ cloves of garlic minced or pressed
1-2 onions chopped

Handful of fresh herbs (oregano, basil, rosemary, thyme, parsley) chopped

Lots of fresh basil (anywhere from 4-8 cups loosely packed leaves)

Olive oil

Sea salt and fresh ground pepper

Steps: Heat the olive oil in a pan and reduce heat to medium-high. Sauté onions, stirring often until they are translucent (about 5 minutes). Then add garlic, stirring frequently for 2 minutes. Next, add the wine if you are using it and wait until the wine has reduced and there is no liquid left. Finally, add the tomatoes and herbs (not basil) and bring to a boil

Simmer on medium-low for at least 45 minutes (you can simmer on low for up to 2 hours). If there is too much liquid and you want a thicker sauce remove some of the liquid with a ladle. Add chopped basil and turn off the heat. Season with salt and pepper to taste.

Moroccan-spiced Lamb

In general, I am an avid vegetable eater, more apt to order a veggie burger than the lamb chops or hamburger. Yet, I gained a serious appreciation for lamb while I was living in Morocco. Specifically, it was a prune and lamb tagine in a small cafe in Tangiers that took me by serious surprise. Since then, I've made some rendition of the dish for every person I've truly loved (and who has caught me at the right time).

I love this recipe for Moroccan lamb because it is flexible. Instead of raisins, you may use prunes, dates, or experiment with figs. If you like a slightly sweeter sauce, you can add even more of the dried fruit. To make this recipe gluten-free, you could use potatoes or tapioca starch to thicken the stew. It is an excellent main dish served with rice, flat bread, potatoes, squash and greens.

Yield: 4 servings

Equipment: Large pot or deep pan

Ingredients for the lamb:

(in order of entry into the dish)
1 small onion
6 cloves of garlic
1 tablespoon paprika
1 teaspoon ground cumin
1 inch piece of fresh ginger
1-2 teaspoons tomato paste (optional)
1 and ½ cup water
8 lamb chops
1 two-inch piece of cinnamon
½ cup raisins
Salt and pepper
Tablespoon or two of flour or other thickening agent (tapioca starch, rice flour, cornstarch)

Steps for the lamb: Defrost the lamb. Heat olive oil in a pan on medium-high and sauté onions for 5 minutes. Reduce heat to medium and add garlic, stirring constantly for 2 minutes. Next, add paprika, ginger, cumin, and stir until aromatic. Then, add the lamb, salt, and pepper, and allow the lamb to brown, turning every few minutes (about 10 minutes total). Add water, tomato paste, cinnamon stick, raisins, then stir and bring to a boil. Reduce to low heat for a slow simmer for about 1 and ½ hours to 2 hours.

Once the lamb is extremely tender, take out 1/2 cup of the liquid and mix it in a bowl with 1-2 tablespoons of flour until the flour dissolves and the mixture is uniform in consistency. Pour the thickened liquid back into the pot with the lamb and allow to simmer at least 5 minutes more.

Taste, adjust the salt and pepper, and serve.

Spaghetti Squash Bake

Who can resist the novelty of the stringy flesh that so delicately mimics spaghetti and works so well to substitute or accompany Italian-style meals. You trade refined wheat for nutrient-packed squash in spaghetti form. I love cooking this squash as the main starch for delicious Italian meals, and to accommodate a culinary experience that is friendly to guests who are gluten-free, paleo, or just hip to the scene.

There are several ways I recommend using this squash to build your main dish: The first is doing the typical, spaghetti and meatballs dish with tomato sauce or other sauce. The second, vegetarian option is to cook the squash and serve a homemade tomato sauce full of greens, garlic, and any other veggies that you have at your disposal. Lastly, you could serve with chicken and another sauce like pesto or mushroom gravy.

Ingredients and steps for the squash:

1 medium sized spaghetti squash, about 2 pounds, or 1000 grams (serves 2-4 if you add enough other protein and veggies).

Cut the squash in half length-wise and scoop out the seeds.

To prepare seeds wash them and get most of the squash flesh off.

Place on foil and spray lightly with oil and salt. Cook at 400° F for 20-30 minutes. While you are baking the squash, make sure to turn over the seeds and mix them around every 7-10 minutes. Place the squash flesh-side down in baking dish. Pour about ½ inch water in the bottom of the dish so that the squash doesn't burn and the heat from the steam allows it to cook more evenly. Bake the squash in the preheated oven at 400° F for about 45 minutes. It is done when the squash is easily dented with your finger, the top is golden, and the flesh forks easily into spaghetti-like strands. Let cool and scoop out the flesh, and serve warm with sauce.

Flexible and Easy Fried Rice

This easy fried rice recipe is a perfect way to use leftover rice, meat and vegetables. It can be made vegetarian and gluten-free, making it a flexible meal to serve for guests with allergies and vegetarian principals. I make this recipe at least once a week, sometimes more. It's great for using up whatever garden veggies I have and any other leftovers (like ground beef, turkey, chicken etc.). You can even add canned salmon or tuna to this. You can make this as veggie stacked as you desire or just put a little in there for color if you are low on produce. I would not try skipping the ginger, garlic, or onion, and especially not the soy sauce and the eggs. Hope you enjoy and make lots of easy fried rice recipes!

Ingredients:

1 cup or so chopped cooked meat (chopped chicken, ground beef, even canned fish, turkey, or just vegetarian)

1.5 – 2 cups cooked rice

Ginger – 1 inch piece peel and chopped into large pieces

Garlic, 1-2 cloves chopped

Chopped veggies (onion, carrot, celery, peppers, cabbage, etc.)

Soy sauce (or gluten-free tamari)

A little maple syrup

Steps: In a large pan, heat olive oil and then add the chopped veggies. Sauté in olive oil until tender (5-10 minutes depending on vegetables).

Add ginger, garlic, and meat, while stirring consistently to avoid burning the garlic for another 3 minutes.

Next, add 1-2 eggs to the pan and stir constantly until cooked, scrambling them in the vegetables. If you need more oil, add it, and then add the rice and stir until heated and combined. Add a few splashes of soy sauce and a small drizzle of maple syrup. Stir until combined, taste, and then add more salt (and/or more soy sauce) and some fresh ground pepper to taste.

Grass-Fed Beef Shepherd's Pie

This recipe for Shepherd's Pie is a favorite among all my dinner guests. It is surprisingly simple to make and requires ingredients that are usually in the home chef's kitchen. It can be made gluten-free and dairy free.

Yield: 4-6 servings

Equipment: large oven safe frying pan or regular frying pan and an oven casserole dish or pie dish

Ingredients for the beef layer:

1-2 pounds grass-fed ground beef (80%-90% fat)

1 medium onion

4 cloves garlic

1-2 large carrots

⅓ cup fresh chopped herbs (thyme, oregano, Cuban oregano, basil, rosemary, sage)

1 cup veggie or other broth
1 teaspoon Worcestershire sauce (optional)
Tomato paste (optional)
Red wine (optional)
Salt and pepper
Ingredients for potato topping:
2-4 large potatoes, cooked
¼ to ½ cup milk (optional)
Salt and pepper to taste (start with about ½ teaspoon salt or less)
Butter is not necessary to make this yummy!

Steps: Sauté onions in olive oil in a large pan until translucent (3 minutes). Add carrots, onions, garlic, and herbs, and sauté a few more minutes over medium-high heat.

Add ground beef and sauté until browned and no longer red, breaking it up as you go. Then add red wine, reduce heat to medium, and let the wine reduce until the aroma of alcohol dissipates and liquid is gone.

After wine has reduced, add broth and optional Worcestershire sauce and let simmer for 10 minutes on medium-high heat until 1/2 of the liquid has been absorbed. At this point, you can thicken the remaining liquid by removing 1/2 cup of it and whisking the tapioca flour in to dissolve it. Then add this back to the pan and simmer for a few minutes.

While the beef is simmering, make the mashed potatoes. If the pan is oven-safe, you may add the mashed potatoes to the top of the beef in the pan and place the whole pan in the oven. Otherwise transfer beef to another oven-safe baking dish and top with the mashed potatoes. Cook for 15-20 minutes at 400° F until the mashed potatoes start to brown and the beef filling begins to bubble. If you like cheese add a layer on top and let it melt for the last few minutes of cooking.

Remove from the oven and let cool for a few minutes before serving with a big green salad.

Baked Chicken and Vegetable Nuggets

Do you remember what you used to like about chicken nuggets or fish sticks? Cross that with eggplant parmesan. This recipe does not require the chicken and veggies to be fried. Instead, they are coated lightly with olive oil and baked. This breaded chicken nugget and veggie recipe is also friendly for gluten-free fans. I use the broken bits of gluten-free bread that I save in the freezer to make a batch of breadcrumbs in the blender. I recommend using high quality chicken, either local, organic or free-range. Conventional chickens are probably the worst of all the meat products in terms of their impact on the environment and the impact on your health.

Yield: serves about 4
Equipment: 2-4 baking sheets and blender
Ingredients:
Sliced chicken breast (4 breast)

Hardcore Health: Live Young!

Eggplant (2 small or 1 large)
Zucchini (2 medium)
1 tablespoon or so olive oil (for the baking pan)
About ¾ cup flour
3 eggs
2-3 cups homemade breadcrumbs (see recipe below)
Optional ½ – 1 cup shredded, hard cheese for adding with bread crumbs (manchego, parmesan, romano, etc.)

Ingredients for bread crumbs:
About 8 slices of left-over bread
1/2 cup of flour (or other flour, try adding oat flour, almond flour, rice flour, spelt flour etc.)
A handful or two of fresh herbs (oregano, basil, rosemary, thyme, etc.)
1/2 to 1 teaspoon salt

Steps: Preheat oven to 375° F and generously oil pan with olive oil. Prepare breadcrumbs by combining breadcrumb ingredients in blender until uniform in size and medium to fine. Place bread crumbs in deep dish (for coating them) and add shredded cheese (optional), save for breading. Coat the sliced chicken, eggplant or zucchini in flour. (For eggplants, it is good to salt them after cutting and before dipping in flour to draw out their water a little)

Dip the chicken and vegetables in whisked egg (let the excess egg drip) and then coat all sides in breadcrumbs. Bake for 10-15 minutes (depending on what and how thick it is) until golden on top and browning on the bottom. Flip and bake another 10-15 minutes until both sides are crispy.

Serve warm with salad, rice, and organic ketchup.

Moroccan Spiced Mahi Mahi and Quinoa

This Moroccan Mahi Mahi recipe is a tribute to my love for Moroccan flavored food. Several years ago I traveled to Morocco twice, and both times I seriously considered staying there because the food was so exotic, warming, spicy, sweet, but still in some ways so simple. I was lucky enough to have a few private cooking lessons with a chef in Azrou, a small town south of Fes. This mahi mahi recipe below is my own creation inspired by my time there. It is a relatively quick way to make an exotic dinner.

Mahi Mahi has become the name for this fish throughout the US. It is also known as dorado or dolphin fish, and it is found in tropical and temperate waters in the Atlantic, Indian, and Pacific Oceans, and the Mediterranean; thus, they also swim in Moroccan waters. They are usually 8-25 pounds.

Servings: 2
Ingredients for the fish:
1 pound Mahi Mahi
1 tsp cumin

1/2 piece inch ginger, chopped fine or grated
1/8 tsp cloves
1/4 tsp cardamom
1/4 tsp coriander
1/8 tsp allspice
2 tbsp olive oil
Salt and pepper to taste
1 onion, chopped
1 medium tomato, chopped roughly
1/4 cup organic white flour

Ingredients for Moroccan quinoa:
1 cup of quinoa (or half quinoa, half rice or millet, or couscous if you want to be traditional)
The juice of 1/2 of a fresh orange
2 cups water or broth
Small handful of raisins
1/2 teaspoon salt or to taste
2 carrots, chopped
2 celery stalks, chopped
1/2 onion, chopped

Steps for the fish: Prepare spices, mixing them together (except ginger). Wash the fish and pat it dry, cut out liver, and make sure there are no bones. Then cut it into large cube size pieces. Place flour on a plate, add a few dashes of salt, and cover pieces of fish in flour.

Now, toast the spices and fresh ginger in a non-stick pan for a few minutes until aromatic. Add the chopped onion and 1 tablespoon olive oil and sauté on low until the onions are translucent.

If you are making the quinoa, start this now and let the onions cook on low (sort of like you are caramelizing them).

Steps for the quinoa: Bring the water to a boil, place all ingredients in a pot and bring to a boil again. Turn to low and simmer for 20 minutes. Remove from heat and leave top on until ready to serve.

When you are ready to start the fish, turn up the heat to medium-high and add another tablespoon of oil and the chopped tomato. Place the fish in the pan and fry/sauté on medium or medium high, flipping them over after 3-4 minutes and cooking for another 3 or 4 minutes. The result should be fish that is somewhat firm and completely cooked inside but still moist, and a saucy, Moroccan spiced tomato mixture that surrounds each piece.

Add more salt and pepper to taste, and serve garnished with chopped fresh mint.

DESSERTS
Baked Bananas Drizzled with Honey

Leave the peel on the banana and slice bananas open, lengthwise.

Place on baking sheet or in baking pan (peel side touching the pan). Then, drizzle the bananas with honey (being careful not to get it all over the pan or the honey will burn).

Bake in oven preheated to 350-400 F for 15 minutes, or until bananas smell aromatic and are slightly browned on top.

Cream Cheese and Walnut Stuffed Dates
Remove the pits from dates. Slice dates in half without cutting it all the way through so that the date "opens". Spread a small amount of cream cheese in the gap and top with a shelled walnut half.

Apples and Honey
Slice apples thin and drizzle a thin amount of pure honey on top. For more calories and protein, add a dab of all natural peanut butter before you top with honey.

Chocolate Avocado Mousse with Banana
For decades of my life, I never really cared for avocados, thinking they were just another bland, fattening, caloric food that people were trending on. But one day, craving chocolate mousse (but abstaining from cow's milk), I came across the avocado mousse concept... and it was this dish that made me LOVE avocados. This recipe is vegan, dairy-free, gluten-free, and uses unrefined sugars. You will have a hard time putting your spoon down.
Yield: 4-6 servings
Equipment: Blender
Ingredients:
Avocados (about 2 large)

1-2 bananas, sliced

¼ -½ cup cocoa powder (depending on the size of the avocadoes)

Honey or maple syrup to taste, or stevia (Ideally the stevia is an addition to honey or maple syrup and allows you to use less of the honey or syrup by adding a few drops of stevia to bring out the sweetness).

Steps: Add avocados and some of the cocoa powder to blender, then add some of the sweetener. Blend until smooth and give it a try. Add more cocoa powder and sweetener to taste. Chill and serve with sliced bananas.

Healthy Oat Flour Banana Bread

This recipe for oat flour banana bread is famous among my family and friends. It is inspired by a recipe on the www.plantoeat.com blog. It is a little bit different than your typical sweet and gooey banana bread. Instead, it is gluten-free and made with simple and healthy ingredients, like coconut oil, and unprocessed sugar, like maple syrup or honey. Its texture is still moist, filling, and it is just sweet enough.

Refined sugar either comes from sugar cane or sugar beets. If the package does not say sugar cane, than you can bet the sugar comes from genetically modified sugar beets. In the refining process, they strip raw sugar of any remaining nutrients. They also use chemical processes to ensure uniform texture, shape, and color, which may result in levels of chemical residue of Phosphoric Acid, Sulfur Dioxide, and Formic Acid in the sugar. In contrast, unrefined sugars are in a more pure form. Usually unrefined sugar comes from sugar cane juice, which is rich in minerals like Phosphorus, Calcium, Iron, Magnesium, and Potassium. In addition, when sugar is refined and processed, there are many harmful ingredients that are added to the sugar as a result. Unrefined natural sweeteners are even better for you than unrefined cane sugar. These have even more nutrients and may require less processing. Maple syrup is my sweetener of choice, but many of my recipes use honey interchangeably with maple syrup. This lends a slightly different, but just as pleasing taste. Other options include: coconut sugar, date sugar, brown rice syrup, molasses, and sucanat.

Yield: 2 bread loaves

Equipment: Blender, 2 bread loaf pans or 1 casserole/brownie pans

Wet ingredients:

6 medium sized and well-ripened bananas

½ cup coconut oil (liquid)

2 eggs (room temperature)

1/4 cup maple syrup (honey, or sugar is ok)

1 teaspoon vanilla

Dry ingredients:

4 cups quick oats (ground in a blender, it equals about 3 cups oat flour)

½ teaspoon salt

1 and ½ teaspoon cinnamon

2 teaspoons baking powder (aluminum free is best for your health)

1 teaspoon baking soda

Steps: Pre-heat the oven to 350° F and coat 2 bread loaf pans with coconut oil. In your blender, pulse quick oats a few times until a flour-like consistency is achieved and measures out to about 3 cups of oat flour. Then, add the rest of the dry ingredients (salt, baking powder, cinnamon) to the blender with the oat flour and pulse a few times to mix.

Pour the dry ingredients from the blender into a medium sized mixing bowl and set aside while you mix the wet ingredients. Then place all wet ingredients into blender. Blend until smooth. Slowly add the wet ingredients to the dry ingredients and mix by hand until incorporated without over-mixing.

Pour batter into pans and place into the oven for about 25-30 minutes, until the banana bread begins to brown on top and a knife or toothpick comes out clean.

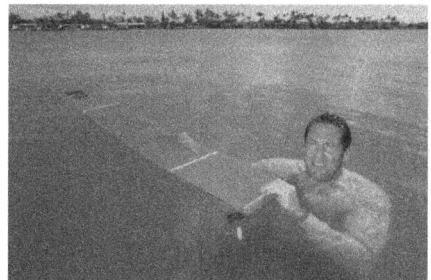

Robert Yonover PhD

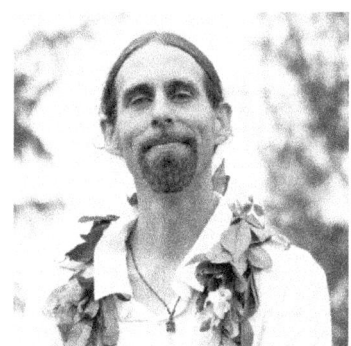

Adam Crowe PDC

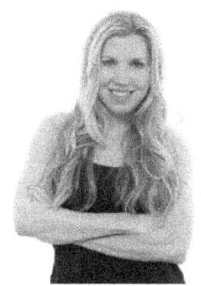

Jennifer Armstrong MS, MD.

www.ingramcontent.com/pod-product-compliance
Lightning Source LLC
Chambersburg PA
CBHW031146020426
42333CB00013B/526